MOODS, EMOTIONS, AND AGING

MOODS, EMOTIONS, AND AGING

Hormones and the Mind-Body Connection

**Phyllis J. Bronson
with Rebecca Bronson**

ROWMAN & LITTLEFIELD PUBLISHERS, INC.
Lanham • Boulder • New York • Toronto • Plymouth, UK

Published by Rowman & Littlefield Publishers, Inc.
A wholly owned subsidiary of The Rowman & Littlefield Publishing Group, Inc.
4501 Forbes Boulevard, Suite 200, Lanham, Maryland 20706
www.rowman.com

10 Thornbury Road, Plymouth PL6 7PP, United Kingdom

British Library Cataloguing in Publication Information Available

Library of Congress Cataloging-in-Publication Data

Bronson, Phyllis J., 1952–
Moods, emotions, and aging : hormones and the mind-body connection / Phyllis J. Bronson with Rebecca Bronson.
p. cm.
Includes bibliographical references and index.
ISBN 978-1-4422-2101-7 (cloth : alk. paper) — ISBN 978-1-4422-2102-4 (electronic)
I. Bronson, Rebecca. II. Title. [DNLM: 1. Hormones—metabolism. 2. Women's Health. 3. Aging—psychology. 4. Mind-Body Therapies. 5. Women—psychology. WP 505]
QP571
612.4'05—dc23
2013004964

Printed in the United States of America

This book is dedicated to Jesse Lawrence Boyce III, my beloved husband, who made the journey worth it all, and to Dwight M. Smith at The University of Denver, my scientific father.

CONTENTS

DISCLAIMER

This book represents reference material only. It is not intended as a medical manual, and the data presented here is meant to assist the reader in making informed choices regarding wellness. This book is not a replacement for treatment(s) that may have been suggested by the reader's personal physician. If the reader believes he or she is experiencing a medical issue, professional medical help is recommended. Mention of particular products, companies, or authorities in this book does not entail endorsement by the publisher or author.

FOREWORD

Dr. Phyllis Bronson brings a unique viewpoint to the subject of bio-identical hormone therapies. Because she has trained as a scientist, she is able to observe the effects of hormones, both the bioidentical and the synthetic analogs, in a dispassionate manner that transcends the current tendencies in medicine to create standards of practice by committee. Each of her clients is a study of one, the real key to creating successful outcomes for each individual.

There is a dimension in this book that is overlooked in most discussions about hormone therapies. This is the importance of the hormones that are created from amino acids, the individual pieces that make up proteins. Dr. Bronson does a careful analysis of each individual for clues to ensure that these amino-acid pieces are plentiful enough to create these other hormones that are so involved in mood, creativity, energy, and sense of self.

Dr. Bronson also explores the dimension of the psyche. She builds on the traditions of psychologists, particularly Jung, and offers her clients the opportunity to explore issues in their present and past life experience. It is a chicken-and-egg dilemma. Can the dysfunctions in relationships lead to hormone imbalances? Can the restoration of hormone balance create the opportunity to solve a trauma or to pave the way to heal a dysfunctional relationship?

Woven into the pattern of this book are the stories of her clients and most importantly, her own story. We are hardwired to empathize and learn from stories. As she tells her own story, she reveals a remarkable discovery. Balancing hormones can make a difference in one's recovery, and interestingly, since she is able to bring her science into stories, she finds that the body seems to demand much more in times of crisis. Little wonder then that many may find in difficult times that their bodies are not able to meet their needs for hormones and to find a path to healing the body and mind.

It may be some time before the medical community starts to address the lack of effectiveness of the one-size-fits-all or flowchart (if this–then that) medicine. This book can serve as a beacon to those who feel that there are better answers that can guide them to demand the changes and the information they need to find their balance.

Carol Peterson, RPh, CNP
Wally Simons, RPh

PREFACE

Descents and Ascents: The Cycles of Life

When I was in my early fifties, I thought I had earned my way to happiness. Although I did not have an easy start to adulthood, I was raised to be very well educated and to do something with my life. Very few women went into the sciences or engineering when I was in college. Women who did often got a clear message that something was wrong with their femininity.

My first marriage was chaotic, and looking back, I can see that it was a choice made while looking for someone to take care of me after my father's sudden and untimely death. While my sister and I were both scientifically inclined, I was first and foremost my "father's daughter." Suddenly, I was thrust into the world without much of a worldly foundation except being my father's daughter, and he was gone. But as I have learned again and again, he left me a legacy of inestimable value, the courage to persevere and to believe in myself. This was the beginning of my journey into adulthood.

As always in my life, skiing was a salvation, and I did a lot of it. I also completed my first degree in chemistry and physics, and I went to work.

My next descent, and what I believed for a long while to be my major midlife crisis, occurred when my first husband returned to his native Canada, leaving me alone with a baby—and not much else, except, once again, myself. I was determined to give my beautiful son, named after my beloved father, the childhood he deserved. For several years, we were alone, my boy and me.

Then I met Jesse, the love of my life. We raised my boy as ours, and Gordon was the joy of our lives together, and we found that rare, extraordinary marriage. We found it, and we were determined to not let anyone hurt it, although people from his past tried.

We were together for eighteen exceedingly happy years, during which time my son grew up into a magnificent young man. Then suddenly, my love, my vital, beautiful Jesse, was diagnosed with stage 4 cancer. He used to hike up Aspen Mountain every morning; he was so strong. But cancer is not selective. It takes what it wants.

I never believed he could die. When treatment with traditional oncology almost killed him, and then gave up on him, we went "outside the box." That is how we discovered Dr. Burzynski, whom I discuss later, and whom I believed extended Jesse's life for a year. However, our private and very expensive insurance company decided that they would not pay for treatment from Dr. Burzynski and for the one biological cancer drug that was truly helping save my husband, leaving us to spend thousands of dollars each month out of pocket for the one drug that this insurance giant claimed was not coded for Jesse's *exact* cancer.

We intended to keep it all going. I would have, and indeed did, go to the ends of the earth to try to save my husband, but then he went downhill.

Then we lost him. I do not remember a thing from the year after losing him. I did what Joyce Carol Oates said the widow must do at the end of her marvelous book *A Widow's Story*—she must survive, and if she did, at the end of that first year, she should congratulate herself, and that is all. I did survive, but I have struggled to regain my sense of life. Of course, our son brings me joy, as do the mountains and my work. Getting this book published is the manifestation for me of the renewal of my life.

Shortly after my husband died, I read Susan Ehrenreich's *Bright-Sided: How the Relentless Promotion of Positive Thinking Has Undermined America*. At the time, I thought how on target she was—sometimes life just happens, and people, even the very best people, get sick and sometimes, yes, they die.

Now, several years into the grief process, I find her book, while intelligently written, is missing something integral to the healing process. I am today much more aligned with the best of Jungian literature as well as some extraordinary books on healing manifestations, such as *Wishes Fulfilled: Mastering the Art of Manifesting* by Wayne Dyer. While I do see how deeply our thinking influences our environment, it is not an exact science. However, to ignore the power of our thinking is as wrong as assuming we can't control anything.

The descent into one's psyche is not a planned, meditative process. As Carl Jung used to say to analysts in training, only when one is utterly flattened can the beginning of the ascent happen. This particular psychology—analytic depth psychology—as Dr. Jung's work is referred to, became a path for me to find my way back to meaning and purpose in life again. Of course, there are other valuable healing discourses; however, this is the journey I am on, and treasure. Thus, it has become pervasive in my work with women and healing the psyche and has become integrated with my biochemical work. For a year I was in a river of grief; the second year became almost harder as I was conscious again, and I realized I had lost what I had lived to be—Jesse's wife. I completely adored him. And because I had done a lot of therapy before I met him, including my first Jungian work, I thought that I was whole and complete when we met. Now I know that I was a work in process, not yet whole. That has come after much grief and work on my own. One is never fully arrived, as we never truly know the future.

During my first marriage, when things started to disintegrate, my husband and I did some couple's counseling with some Jungian therapists he had met. On our first visit, when I was asked what I thought the purpose of marriage is, I responded, "Well, I think he is supposed to make me happy." This was definitely the wrong answer to give a Jungian analyst! I was immediately assigned to read *The Wounded Woman: Healing the Father-Daughter Relationship* by Linda Schierse Leonard.

My former husband decided that the problems in our marriage were mine—so I should go to couple's therapy alone, and I did. He was wrong; the deepest healing happens with the couple. I started to learn about dreams and the unconscious. My life was in upheaval; I was trying to make a marriage that I no longer believed in work. I did not want to live in Canada; I wanted to raise my boy in Colorado. I realize now that this time was a gift, as painful as it was. I was starting to learn to trust my instinctive life. This is separate from my scientific life, and I am passionate about each. I had a dream, over and over, of an airplane flying between narrow canyons, trying to break free into the open sky. Finally it did, and so did I. I left my husband, returned to Aspen, and worked hard.

Then I met Jesse, and eighteen years of inestimable joy later, he died. The thing that saved my life these past two years was finding a superlative male therapist to do grief work with. We survived the two years of the nigrato (descent) into the journey of grief together when I felt numb. Only recently as I write this has my unconscious started to slowly show me the way back to life. I am now in a period of latency— meaning waiting. In her book *The Cat: A Tale of Feminine Redemption*, Marie-Louise von Franz, another great analyst, says women must learn the way of the cat—that sometimes watching and waiting is all we must do, not acting until right action reveals itself to us.

I write all of this as a backdrop to let you know that I know something about midlife crisis. The one I am just emerging from is the true one: all prior thoughts that I had about midlife were mere intellectual attempts to live from what I have told women for years they must do at midlife: "Learn to hang out with uncertainty."

Now, I can truly say that I have become the living embodiment of that. I am slowly renewing my life, and I see the germs of the creative process sprouting. I no longer wake up in total fear about how to make life work, but rather I am invested in finding meaning and purpose once again. I was tested this past year when I experienced betrayal by a colleague I had done a lot for. I naively assumed that while I was down, and away caring for my husband, he would be more supportive, not less.

I have been in the desert. I have looked at my psyche from every angle. I accept responsibility for my mistakes; I feel remorse that I was not better prepared to face life alone even though I thought I was. I know our son will have the future he deserves, and I will make these days up to him.

So with my life upside down, how do I invent the future? By taking it one day at a time and not getting out of bed until I am aligned with my higher self—and I do that frequently throughout the day—and remember who I am. When I start to feel sad or negative, I shift the energy to a state of feeling as much relief as possible. I feel as good as I can and come from that, rather than hoping to get there.

INTRODUCTION: WOMEN AND THEIR MOODS

What is not brought to consciousness comes to us as Fate.

—C. G. Jung

HORMONES, MOOD, AND MIND/BODY INTEGRATION

I woke up this morning feeling flat and agitated, without my usual optimism. This is how many of my clients tell me they often feel. Then I realized I had not used any hormones for twenty-four hours: bioidentical topical (cream) hormones need to be used twice a day—after twelve hours, there is little left in the body. I was in the shower thinking about my bad mood, got out, and used the compounded cream. Within fifteen minutes I felt an immense lift to my mood and was able to start the day in the right space. Although I know from my own research that transdermal estrogen is a great mood elevator and can work in as little as ten minutes, experiencing this firsthand was an eye-opener for me. Many menopausal and younger women live in this constant state of agitation and/or depression, and they cannot see any way out. My purpose in writing this book is quite simple. I did some of the most important early research defining why bioidentical hormones (notably progesterone) are so important for women's health and how these hormones differ from synthetic drugs. I want to enlighten women and their doctors to new information on this subject and to give women the information they need in order to age with grace and health and happiness.

My work is in the field of orthomolecular medicine and chemistry, which seeks to define the impact of hormones and nutrients on mood and emotion. My colleagues and I have been studying hormonal-based mood disorders for many years, and our approach is different from that of traditional medicine. Orthomolecular medicine is a nutrition- and biochemistry-based approach founded by two-time Nobel Prize winner Linus Pauling. Orthomolecular practitioners look for vitamin, mineral, amino acid, and hormonal imbalances in the body as the basis of psychological, emotional, and physical problems. They then use biogenic substances—that is, substances already naturally existing in the body—to offset imbalances and deficiencies. In my work, I apply this mind/body strategy to correct distortions in brain chemistry and hormones that lead to intense mood problems. I focus on the core of where women live: their emotional world, helping women to understand the connection between their changing hormone levels (throughout their lives) and their moods.

My research deals with real women who know that life is full of challenges. I hear over and over again that smart woman are not on a quest for perfection but rather want the ability to live well through the passages of life. This is where natural (bioidentical) hormones can be extraordinarily helpful. Proper use of real hormones, those that mimic what is native to us as women, can help to ease the transitions of life and aging by making women feel more optimistic and vital.

THE TRADITIONAL APPROACH

For years the standard practice in gynecology was to put women on hormone replacement therapy (HRT) as they approached menopause. Then in July of 2002 a huge hormonal study known as the Women's Health Initiative (WHI) Study was abruptly halted, due to observations that women on these drugs were developing varying degrees of pathology. Unfortunately, the study was flawed from the outset in that a statistically relevant number of the women in the study had hypertension, diabetes, or were obese, although this was not noted at the time. This was further complicated by the fact that the majority of the women started on HRT well past the onset of menopause, averaging ten to fifteen years. Scientists now know that major aspects of aging happen at the time of menopause and are much more difficult to rectify later.

The Women's Health Initiative Study had two components: Prempro® for women with intact ovaries and uteruses (terminated in July 2002), and Premarin® only for women who had had hysterectomies (terminated in March 2004). The Prempro study showed an increase in breast cancer in approximately 2.5 percent of women; this was not considered statistically relevant. The study rightly was stopped, but not for the right reasons. Since 1997, the scientific community has known that Provera® synthetic progestin—not real progesterone—has had negative implications on the female cardiovascular system because it decreases vascular function.[1, 2] The Premarin-only study data showed no increased risk of breast cancer or heart attacks but a very slight increased risk of stroke for women over sixty.[3]

Perhaps the biggest flaw in this study (and the most misunderstood) is that "hormones" come in different forms. This particular study was performed with synthetic hormones—that is, hormones manufactured by a pharmaceutical company. On farms in North Dakota and Canada, mares are impregnated and then confined from the fourth month to the eleventh month of pregnancy. During this time, their urine is collected, and the urine estrogens are packed into pills. *Premarin* is a condensation of the words *pregnant mares' urine*. This urine contains estradiol and mostly estrone, a more toxic form of estrogen, along with equilin, a horse estrogen that never occurs in humans. These are known as "conjugated estrogens." And Prempro contains medroxyprogesterone, which is progesterone that has been chemically modified in a laboratory so as to make it patentable. "Bioidentical" hormones are considerably different from the synthetic ones used in this study, and these hormones do not have the usual side effects of their synthetic cousins. Much of my research at the University of Denver with Dwight Smith, PhD, has been devoted to understanding the differences between synthetic and bioidentical hormones, and these differences are substantial. Dr. Smith is my great mentor, colleague, and scientific "father." I owe him an enormous intellectual debt. He is the former chair of the chemistry department and the former chancellor of the University of Denver, and his brilliant approach to molecular science has been the basis of much that I have evolved into as a scientist. Unfortunately, because of the side effects and the bad outcome of the study, *all* hormones were given a bad reputation, and women became scared to use them.

Another study, the Women's Health Initiative Memory Study (WHIMS), showed that women using conjugated equine estrogens (from horse urine) plus MPA (medroxyprogesterone acetate), a synthetic progestin, had an increase in dementia over a five-year period. My research showed that there are significant chemical differences between the synthetic progestin (used in this study) and "natural" progesterone made by the human body and/or compounding pharmacies. These chemical differences have an impact on the way that the molecules function in the body. Unfortunately, other aspects of these large, randomized studies have overshadowed this information.

It is important to note that some versions of hormones produced by standard pharmaceutical companies are actually bioidentical in their structures: Estrace® and Prometrium® come to mind, as well as Vivelle® patches.

When the Women's Health Initiative was released and halted in 2002, it set off a wave of misinformation that has permeated the field ever since. First, many women were told by their doctors to stop hormone replacement therapy (HRT). So they did. Many women started feeling lousy without their hormones. Inquisitive physicians observed this, and over time they started reintroducing estrogen back to women at high risk for depression and heart disease and at low risk for potential complications of estrogen. These complications were largely due to synthetic combination hormones, although many doctors did not understand this.

I first started researching hormones and their impact on the female brain in 1995. This has evolved into my seminal work on the mood biochemistry of women at midlife and beyond. I have completed original research in this area, both from a molecular biochemical basis and a clinical approach. My academic work has been carefully integrated into our clinical work in the biochemistry of mood disorders that I conduct in Aspen, Colorado. For many years, I partnered with the late Harold Whitcomb, MD, and upon his retirement in the year 2000 I have worked with other physicians, notably Chris Martinez, MD, in Aspen, and others around the globe. Many traditionally trained doctors had never heard of bioidentical hormones, or hormones that did not come from pharmaceutical giants such as Wyeth, the maker of the synthetic hormones Premarin and Provera.

The majority of women we worked with felt great when they started on real (bioidentical) progesterone. Various physicians around the United States and abroad began looking at the research I was doing and wanted to introduce this into clinical practice. I had a rare opportunity to integrate scientific and clinical work. Patients experienced an increase in well-being, as well as a decrease in the agitation that is dominant in many women as they approach midlife. Although they did not know why, they knew it felt right.

WHAT WOMEN TELL US

Getting older is hard on the female psyche; women struggle to hold on to what they have: their looks, their men, and their joy. It seems harder for women than for men because women so often feel at the effect of the males in their lives and the unconscious domination—even from good men—that women feel within their own secret selves.

We see an array of books on women's health, many of them written by people with little or no scientific background. Often, the authors are celebrities who have already gathered a large audience, and they are talking about a hot topic that brings these books rapidly into the mainstream. This can present a problem for women, as they are being bombarded by misinformation about a topic that is already confusing. How does one sort out the "good" information from the myths?

After its publication in 2006, *The Female Brain* by Louann Brizendine, MD, set off a wave of interest. The book discussed differences between men and women in the context of mood issues, and it was a historical account of the importance of estrogen. In response to the halting of the Women's Health Initiative, Brizendine wrote, "Many scientists now believe that HT (hormone therapy) should be thought of as a protector against age-related brain decline, although this belief conflicts with the findings of the WHI." In her book she quotes Fred Naftolin of Yale University: "So . . . these menopausal symptoms are warnings of estrogen deficiency that are singing out to alert us of the need to test the idea of prevention by timely estrogen treatment."

While this was interesting and enlightening to both men and women, the book did not provide women with new information that they could use in their lives. However, a number of women contacted us after reading the book, looking for ways to take estrogen again. Unfortunately, Brizendine did not make the distinction between real progesterone and progestins, the crux of what went wrong with the Women's Health Initiative.

Celebrity Suzanne Somers writes about bioidentical hormones in her books, and although this has provided a springboard for doctors to begin to look at these issues, some of what she says is misleading. Somers's celebrity status has allowed her to make a contribution by waking up both women and the medical establishment to the importance of bioidentical hormones. Her books, however, tend to oversimplify an incredibly complicated field. As a result, those who most need to hear it ignore the message.

Her premise, that women should take so much estrogen that they get their periods again, is not a good idea for women. In cultures in which women are more frequently pregnant and nursing, causing them to menstruate less frequently, there is far less female cancer. This may be linked to the fact that extreme rising and falling of primary estrogen (estradiol), as happens when a woman is cycling regularly, is stimulating and not good for the endometrium (lining of the uterus). By not using progesterone for two weeks to a month, women will "have a period." This is not a period. A woman menstruates when she is ovulating and could therefore become pregnant. This is not what is happening with sixty-year-old women on this protocol. They are having breakthrough bleeding induced by the withdrawal of progesterone, which causes the endometrial tissue to shed and bleed. Further, it is incorrect that women are simulating a pregnancy state by using physiologic doses of hormones. During pregnancy, the levels of estrogen and progesterone in a woman's body are enormously high; the levels recreated by using bioidentical hormones properly simply help women get back to balance. Many women have told me how bad they felt and how much agitation and anxiety recurred when they stopped progesterone completely, even for a short while.

Using hormones as part of a quest for the "fountain of youth" is not good medical practice. Rather, they should be used to enhance the aging process. Telling women that if they use massive doses of estradiol (primary estrogen) that they will become youthful is misleading and wrong. This kind of transcendent approach to aging and to life is harmful—it is wrong to suggest that aging is unnecessary and irrelevant. Women, generally, do not want to look thirty-five at sixty-two; they want to age gracefully and without concurrent aches and pains.

In my office, when we talk about mood and emotion, there appears to be a "never done" aspect to female processing. Women sometimes live in their relational world, and it can make it much harder for them to "compartmentalize" the way men do. A man's emotional world may be falling apart, or seeming to, and yet often he remains stoic, able to get work done, to function seemingly seamlessly. It can be different for women. They can feel as if they are drowning in sorrow or bursting open with rage.

Women must develop the ability to accept themselves at any age. The shallowness of Western media in the movies, for example, glorifies shallow thinking in general. Rational, thinking women are a threat to the general herd mentality of some people, and sometimes this can be a threat to their own marriages. We have so many women tell us that by containing the vast emotional-hormonal sea with a good balance of hormones and nutrients (vitamins, minerals, amino acids) and by learning to work with one's own thoughts, one can live in a state of joy at midlife and beyond.

I

IN DEFENSE OF ESTROGEN

The story of the aging female has taken on a life of its own in the Western world today. Yet the most basic academic aspects of how to slow down the aging process are shunned, often in the quest of the "addiction to perfection."[1] Some women seek to numb their wrinkles and have plastic surgery for every flaw. But these therapies are bandages serving only to cover up their aging bodies.

Life can become harder as we age, and the choices we face do not seem as limitless as they once did. Were they ever really that way, or was that simply the perception of youth? Aging gives us a sense that the walls are closing in, and traditional medicine, despite all its great capabilities, does not help people develop coping skills and more honest ways of looking at transitional times. Often, illness shows up in times of great uncertainty, as the person takes on the stress of change at a biological level. While joy is a great container for health, despair is a box for illness. Learning to tolerate uncertainty is the great challenge of this midlife transition time. Some people do it well, and some fall by the wayside, succumbing to many things such as divorce, serious illness, or depression. These events can take people out—or make them grow in unexpected ways. Unfortunately, much of traditional Western medicine (especially cancer medicine) is fear based, promoting fear and toxic thinking in many people and causing them to give up.

I see a great deal of sorrow in women. Many are alone and have given up on finding a life partner to grow older with. Others are in unhealthy marriages, and they are holding on, seemingly for dear life.

Once in this state, they cannot thrive, and neither can their relationships. These women need a great deal of support, both biochemically and psychologically, to move through this midlife passage. Women and men in healthy relationships need support as well, because the frontiers of relationship are changing as we age and in the times we live in, and nothing is certain. In fact, learning to tolerate uncertainty is one of the big challenges for healthy aging.

HORMONES AND AGING

Menopause is defined by hormonal changes, and for some women the precipitous drop in estrogen can be emotionally overwhelming. All women experience a significant drop in estrogen as they approach midlife some time in their late forties, usually before menopause, and this hormone plays a major role in aging. In the early 1900s, women entered menopause at about age fifty—which was about their life expectancy. In the last hundred years, the average woman's life expectancy has increased by three decades, meaning that she can expect to spend about thirty years of her life postmenopausal. There is no precedence for this transition into the midlife years, or indeed, into older age. Concurrent with this increase in life expectancy (and perhaps as a result of it), over the past fifty years menopause has become a medical condition and is being treated as such by both the pharmaceutical industry and the medical establishment. About sixty years ago, the medical establishment told women approaching menopause to take estrogen. The first widely marketed synthetic oral estrogens made for the purpose of hormone replacement therapy (HRT) in the United States were distributed in the 1940s. This worked for about twenty-five years, until women who were taking estrogen began to develop endometrial problems (a thickening of the lining of the uterus). To counteract this tendency to build too thick a uterine lining, the medical establishment decided that women also needed progesterone, and the pharmaceutical industry again stepped in with synthetic progestins. Doctors were told that women needed "progestins" to protect them from endometrial problems. This was a catastrophe for women because the synthetic progestins produced some major detrimental side effects, most notably a potential for cardiac problems and a profound negative impact on mood. What women actually needed was real progesterone to balance excess endogenous (internal) or exogenous (added) estrogen, and still allow estrogen to do its work on mood and health.

ESTROGEN: FRIEND OR FOE?

Women are profoundly affected by fluctuations in their hormones, both natural as well as those from exogenous sources such as birth control pills and hormone replacement therapy (HRT). In 2002, after the Women's Health Initiative (WHI) was halted due to safety concerns, the medical establishment largely recommended that doctors take women off their hormones. Women, particularly those vulnerable to depression and related mood issues, knew they did not do well without their hormones, notably estrogen, but they had no place to turn.[2]

Estrogen in the female human is a composite of three molecules produced by our bodies: estrone (E1), estradiol (E2), and estriol (E3). Estradiol is the most potent form of estrogen and makes up about 10 percent of the estrogen produced by the ovaries.

Estrone (E1) is twelve times weaker in terms of biological impact and also makes up about 10 percent of a woman's normal estrogen levels; however, it is considered to be a potentially more dangerous form of estrogen, and in fact it may be the principal culprit in estrogen toxicity. Amazingly, E1 is the major estrogen in Premarin, still the biggest-selling pharmaceutical estrogen in the world even today. Until recently it was assumed that estrone was synthesized from estradiol primarily in the liver, and there was a biological balance between these two estrogens. The current understanding is that as women age, they produce a great deal of estrone in their fat cells (and many women gain weight and have bigger fat cells as they age). Thus, postmenopausal women naturally produce more estrone, even as their more important estrogen or estradiol is decreasing.[3]

As the less desirable estrogen, E1, rises as we age, the vitality-enhancing estrogen, E2, decreases, and brain fog and depression often set in. These are two of the first signs of serious estrogen imbalance.

Estradiol (E2) is a critical molecule for the aging female and acts as a defense against depression and loss of cognitive function. A wealth of data suggest that if E2 supplementation is started at the proper age it has profound, beneficial effects on all aspects of a woman's biology, including moods and emotion, heart disease, memory, bone density, and cancer risk. Even Alzheimer's disease may be slowed or halted due to regulatory mechanisms on beta amyloid protein; this is the toxic protein that builds up in early Alzheimer's disease.

Estriol (E3) is the weakest form of estrogen, and although it is eighty times weaker than estradiol it makes up about 80 percent of a woman's total estrogen. Estriol is produced from estrone in a complex chemical reaction and appears to counterbalance estrone's toxicity: Asian women who eat a diet high in fermented soy products have higher levels of estriol and appear to have less cancer, leading researchers to believe that estriol somehow plays a "protective role," possibly by creating less toxic metabolites.[4]

Many women have relied on bioidentical replacement hormones that are prescribed by their doctors and formulated in compounding pharmacies. These are small, independent pharmacies that make up hormone formulations specified to the woman's individual needs. The substances are FDA approved, and the doses are geared to individual women. These hormones are biologically identical to those that are produced in the human body. Estriol is one of these hormones, and in January of 2008, the U.S. Food and Drug Administration ordered pharmacies to stop providing bioidentical estriol, stating that it was a "new and unapproved drug" and that its "safety and effectiveness was unknown." This is not so, since bioidentical estriol has been in use for years, though not in a pharmaceutical patented form.[5]

In a press conference, the FDA admitted that no *adverse event involving compounded bioidentical estriol has ever been reported.* Research involving fifteen thousand women funded by the Department of Defense and conducted at Kaiser Permanente Oakland found that women who produced the most estriol during their first pregnancy were 58 percent less likely to develop breast cancer over the next forty years. Estriol is a major estrogen throughout a woman's reproductive years, and it soars to enormous levels (up to a thousand times) during pregnancy.[6]

How can bioidentical estriol, identical to every woman's natural estriol, be unsafe or ineffective? And how can the FDA claim that a substance present in our bodies from the dawn of humanity is a "new and unapproved drug"? It's hard to find answers to these questions, even as many women wait for such solutions to the ups and downs of menopause.

LOW ESTROGEN AND BRAIN FOG

Research has shown that hormone replacement can have multiple benefits relating to cognition and general brain function, and it appears that neurological changes can be correlated with declines in estrogen levels. In particular, scientists have investigated whether a decrease in 17-beta estradiol might be predictive of the onset of clinical depression in vulnerable women. There is increasing evidence that the decline of 17-beta estradiol in perimenopausal and menopausal women precipitates the general feeling of malaise and lack of well-being that many women experience in midlife.

Michelle came to my office saying she was afraid she was developing early Alzheimer's. At age forty-six, she felt as if she was in a dense fog that seemed to set in every day after lunch. It was present in the morning as well, although it was not as bad. Her periods were still regular, and she had no other obvious symptoms of menopause.

When gynecologists look at fertility patterns, they measure circulating blood hormone levels during the first part of a woman's menstrual cycle. In my work examining mood changes, I measure hormone levels at the time of the month when women feel the worst—that is, during the progesterone, or luteal, phase of the cycle, which is the latter phase. Women like Michelle, who have a history of cyclical depression, often feel well only in the early phase of their monthly cycle, usually days seven to fourteen, when estrogen rises toward ovulation. Michelle's bloodwork was therefore done at day twenty-one, during the second ovulatory peak, after the first peak at ovulation around day fourteen.

Even though Michelle was still menstruating, her estrogen and progesterone had greatly declined, and she was in late perimenopause at age forty-six. Because the external symptoms had just recently appeared, she thought this had happened quickly; however, these symptoms are generally years in the making. Initially, progesterone declines, with a resultant anxiety and irritability. When estradiol starts its descent, the fall is more rapid, and the negative effect on women's moods and emotions is often staggering.

When a woman starts supplementing with bioidentical primary estrogen, otherwise known as E2 or estradiol, the resultant increase in her well-being can happen quite rapidly. This supplementation can be in the form of a pharmaceutical such as a patch or part of a compounded transdermal cream (our preference). Unlike bioidentical transdermal progesterone that is only available through compounding pharmacies, there are other bioidentical forms of estrogen available at the drugstore. Unfortunately, the most common forms of estrogen are derived from horse urine (not bioidentical for humans) and contain mostly E1 or estrone, the least desirable estrogen. The first time Michelle applied transdermal cream of bioidentical estrogen, her brain fog lifted within one hour.

Transdermal means "absorbed through the skin," and this is the preferred choice of hormone delivery, as I believe it allows for the fewest side-chain metabolites that can be deleterious and the transdermal delivery most closely mimics the circadian and natural rhythms of one's own hormonal uptake. These transdermal, bioidentical hormones are made by prescription at compounding pharmacies.

The creams that are applied to the skin are biologically compatible and are in an oil base, so that they can be safely and well absorbed through the skin into the portal blood. At my practice, we use this form much more than pills or patches, as it is more consistent with the way in which hormones are processed internally. Further, doctors now resuming the use of estrogen will often use patches, believing they are the same as bioidentical creams. The Vivelle patch is primarily estradiol. This is certainly better than Premarin, which is made from horse urine and is not bioidentical, but the problem with patches, injectibles, and oral delivery is that the hormones are not delivered in the rhythms natural to the female's own patterns but rather in a steady stream. There are bioidentical forms of these various delivery systems, often from regular pharmacies, and some compounding pharmacies make the injected pellets. I do not recommend them, nor do my closest, most highly regarded medical and scientist colleagues. Additionally, because the estrogen patch also does not include estriol (E3), we believe this may be an important safety factor. The creams I work with contain both E2 (estradiol) and E3 (estriol). These hormones are absorbed almost instantly and are never stored in fat cells. This is not even in the realm of possibility, as they are designed to be microdispersed in an oil base that is metabolized as a fat as soon as it hits the bloodstream. I have seen and recorded significant and rapid changes in E2 levels to document the efficacy of this approach.

SOME CASE STUDIES

Libby had a curvy body typical of women who are estrogen dominant, and she had struggled with body image issues all her adult life. She had a tendency toward obsession and anxiety—now she felt quite down, which was new territory for her. She had elevated cholesterol and signs of early menopause. Her estradiol level (a critical marker in our work) had dropped by more than 25 percent in six months. This is so important: some women do fine for years at a certain relatively low set point. Other women such as Libby are used to much higher, naturally occurring levels of estrogen, so when it drops precipitously the impact is great. She started on a statin drug; one of seven that are heavily prescribed by doctors to help lower cholesterol.

She probably did not need this drug, although the cardiologist she saw uses them a lot and is so dogmatic almost no one dares argue with him. She needed lifestyle and diet changes, supplements, and estrogen. She loved eggs, which while nutrient dense are very also very high in arachidonic acid, a proinflammatory molecule. She also ate a lot of hamburgers because her boys loved them and she ate what she fixed them. We recommend that women lean toward more of a plant-based approach to eating. As mentioned earlier, there are many phytoestrogens in the plant and vegetable world that help counter toxic environmental factors.

A meta-analysis published in 2011 of thirty-four thousand patients showed that patients with various risk factors such as elevated cholesterol, hypertension, but no heart disease were at low risk of heart attack and stroke. The drug companies making the statins funded all but one of the fourteen studies included.

While it was clear from this study that statins did reduce the risk of cardiovascular events, there were major flaws in the study. For people at low risk it was reported that "1,000 people would have to be treated with statins for one year to reduce deaths from 9 to 8." Many people in the study reported side effects such as muscle pain, unexplained memory loss, and confusion.

Libby was not a high-risk, potential cardiac patient. My colleague who treated her later said estrogen could have done more for her from the outset because she clearly had signs of significant estrogen depletion. This was not an aging woman: she was only forty-six when her first physician, a cardiologist, put her on a statin. Usually, heart disease in women occurs after menopause. Often changes in heart patterns such as palpitations are connected to hormonal fluctuations. Further, estrogen decreases levels of LDL (low-density lipoprotein, also known as the bad cholesterol), and raises HDL—the good cholesterol. Estrogen therapy lowers cardiovascular risk, but not when supplied with a synthetic progestin as was done in the first phase of the Women's Health Initiative. Because of this, much confusion has developed.

After about a week of starting a statin drug, Libby complained of feeling disconnected and confused. This is not uncommon, as some people report extreme memory lapses when on these drugs. After about three weeks, she developed a sense of "feeling weird"; significantly one day she could not find her way home and her husband became alarmed.

Her hormone panel revealed an astonishingly low level of estradiol for a forty-six-year-old, still-menstruating woman: less than 20 pg, at day twenty-one of her cycle. (It is common for us to look at day twenty-one of the cycle when we are looking at mood issues. As we are not examining fertility patterns, we are focused on when most women start to have emotional or cognitive symptoms.) Her doctor weaned her off the statin and put her on a compounded cream of estrogen and progesterone; her confusion was what is known as iatrogenic—inadvertently induced by a drug protocol that is not working for a given patient.

The unpublicized part of the halted 2002 Women's Health Initiative Study is that for women like Libby, not getting the estrogen they need leads to some pretty dire consequences. She actually thought she was losing her memory—suddenly, and seemingly inexplicably, until the dots were connected. Her symptoms cleared rapidly once starting the cream hormones. Initially, she used an extra dose of estrogen midday if the vagueness came on after lunch, which had been the case, and after a few weeks she rarely needed that.

The following case study illustrates how not to approach estrogen deficiency. A woman, Mary, whom I saw years ago, would only use progesterone, as she considered herself a "disciple" of John Lee, MD, who had raised the veil on the critical importance of progesterone in his books, such as *What Your Doctor May Not Tell You about Menopause* and others. His books were wonderful, and remain classics, but in his quest to teach women about the importance of progesterone he missed something vital: that progesterone is the secondary molecule for women, after estrogen. When I saw this woman about fifteen years ago, she had signs and symptoms of cognitive decline. My partner at the time was one of very few physicians questioning pharmaceutical synthetic hormones. He told Mary that she needed both estrogen and progesterone. I agreed, and we discussed how progesterone's role is twofold: to balance excess estrogen in the body and offset side effects, and to promote calm in the female psyche. She said she only wanted the calmness, and she refused to consider the facts that were especially relevant for someone with early cognitive decline. She was then in her late forties. She did not return to us professionally except to get a prescription for more progesterone. My partner gave this to her, as he considered it better than nothing in terms of protection, which it certainly was. But in terms of cognition, I now believe that if progesterone is used solely when estrogen is in serious decline as in a case such as this, that symptoms will get worse. And that is what has happened.

Mary has been all over the world looking for help from various doctors and other healers. She is also someone I see socially once in a while, and every time I see her she looks drier and drier and seems vaguer and vaguer. She is a lovely woman by nature, and this is sad to witness; however, I am also astounded. I do seminal research with hormones, and she has not once, in over ten years, asked me a single question. I know that primary estrogen, estradiol, could alleviate 80 percent of the brain fog within hours, and this is her dominant concern. She is now taking a drug generally used for older people with Alzheimer's, which she claims she does not have. The data on the real potential of these drugs known as cholinesterase inhibitors is dismal, because there is only evidence of minimal improvement, which does not last very long, yet doctors write millions of dollars of prescriptions for them and the general public downs them trustingly, willingly. The latest data show them to only slightly halt cognitive decline for six to twelve months.[7]

The basic premise of my work of is that "women are not allergic to their own biology!" So much faith in medicine is lost daily by an approach that puts a new protocol or drug on a pedestal one week and knocks it off shortly later. So often women have told me that they felt they could not be open or honest with various physicians; this happened frequently following the halting of the 2002 Women's Health Initiative Study. Women were so flooded with fear based on erroneous conclusions from flawed data that hormones became truly a study in throwing out the baby with the bath water. I saw mature, sophisticated women give up their estrogen . . . and fall apart; those vulnerable to flat-affect depression suffering the most.

My journey during the past decade as a woman scientist involved in the controversial field of hormone therapy has been difficult at times. I have, over these ten years, often found myself between two extremes: on the one hand, receiving accolades from scientific and open-minded medical colleagues, and on the other, anger from medical doctors who were ignorant of the science or who did not want to know anything different than what they had been taught in medical school. I have seen the subject of bioidentical hormones bashed on various pop news shows, not scientific programming. I found that many medical colleagues had difficulty with science that was "outside the box" and original. Nowhere is this more prominent than in the manufacture of synthetic hormones for women, from puberty through menopause.

Why not instead open a discourse on the vast gray areas in medicine? This would provide a giant leap forward and allow women to enjoy far more healthful and balanced lives.

2

THE TRUTH ABOUT PROGESTERONE

THE MOLECULE OF CALM

> Rage and bitterness do not foster femininity. They harden the heart and make the body sick.
>
> —Marion Woodman

Natural progesterone is the forgotten hormone, or the never discovered hormone, depending on one's point of view. Progesterone is a specific hormone, and progestin refers to a class of compounds (generally synthetically made) that can sustain the endometrium (uterine lining) and prevent ovulation. Because of this, progestins are a major component of most birth control pills. Progesterone, like estrogen, is made in the ovaries during the menstrual cycle.

The effects of natural progesterone have been overlooked because of the emphasis on estrogen, and this oversight has had unfortunate consequences. Natural progesterone protects against breast cancer, while estrogen increases the risk of breast and endometrial cancer if not used in conjunction with natural progesterone, because estrogen stimulates cellular proliferation. Progesterone stimulates the formation of osteoblasts and thus promotes the production of new bone. Estrogen does not produce new bone, although it does help to retard bone loss. According to John Lee, MD, estrogen unopposed by progesterone leads to an imbalance in hormone regulation. The relevant symptoms are fibrocystic breasts, uterine fibroids, and endometrial and breast cancer.[1]

In 1994, a study led by the National Institutes of Health called the Women's Health Initiative (WHI) was started with the hope of establishing that the synthetic drugs Premarin and Provera would relieve menopause symptoms, and go further by protecting aging women from heart attacks, strokes, osteoporosis, and cancer. However, the study (which was halted early for safety reasons) proved unequivocally that the drugs were *unsafe* and were significant factors in increasing the risk of heart attacks, strokes, and breast cancer in the more than sixteen thousand women studied. This led doctors to take millions of women off Premarin, Prempro, and Provera overnight. Predictably, these women started to feel horrible in the aftermath of the drugs' sudden withdrawal, and their physicians told them there were no alternatives. Instead they prescribed antidepressants or birth control pills with shoddy results.

One year after this disaster, the American College of Obstetrics and Gynecology developed new guidelines that encouraged physicians to prescribe the same drugs in lower doses for shorter periods of time. Yet, and this is key, the safety of this "low dose option" was *never* proven scientifically. Why would the wrong substance be acceptable just in a lower dose?

Meanwhile, many conventional physicians have ignored the effectiveness of bioidentical or natural progesterone, which is formulated to be identical to the progesterone molecule that is produced by the human body. There are twenty-five years of scientific research with hundreds of studies in the United States and Europe that have demonstrated that bioidentical hormones, estradiol and micronized progesterone, are equally or more effective than synthetics—and safer.

Holtorf Medical Group has reviewed hundreds of peer-reviewed articles and studies and found that bioidentical hormones were associated with lower risks, including the risk of breast cancer and cardiovascular disease, and they were more effective than their synthetic and animal-derived counterparts.[2]

In a European study, the data indicated that adverse effects of HRT may have been dependent on a variety of factors, including the estrogen and progesterone/progestin formulation, dosage, mode of administration, patient's age, associated diseases, and duration of treatment. All estrogen formulations and modes of administration had similar beneficial effects on vasomotor and urogenital symptoms and on bone structure. But cardiovascular and invasive breast cancer risks were higher with oral estrogen than with transdermal estradiol, and they were also *higher with many progestin compounds than with micronized (bioidentical) progesterone.*[3] Yet mainstream medicine has buried its head in the sand and refused to take these studies seriously.

NATURAL PROGESTERONE VERSUS SYNTHETIC PROGESTERONE

Most women and their gynecologists are not well informed about the immense value of bioidentical (real) progesterone and do not know that there is a difference between real progesterone and synthetic progestins (a lab-invented form of progesterone used in birth control pills and hormone replacement therapy [HRT], among other medications). As part of my graduate dissertation, I did work comparing synthetic progestins to natural (bioidentical) progesterone. Although the pharmaceutical companies would have you believe that these chemicals are the same, they are biochemically quite different, and the differences at a molecular level cause them to react differently in the human body. Synthetic progestins are the drug makers' fantasy progesterone. While these molecules are progesterone "look-alikes" and have the same goal in mind (mediating effects of estrogen on proliferative tissue, such as the endometrium), in fact they are not progesterone. These pharmaceutical mimics are like duplicate keys that will fit in the lock but not unlock the door. You may wonder why the drug companies even bothered to produce these in the first place, and herein lies the basis of one of Western medicine's darkest sides. Since these drugs are not the same as those hormones produced in the female body, they are patentable, while naturally occurring substances are not. Thus, there is the potential for huge financial gain for the pharmaceutical companies.

Dr. Jeffery Dach, an eminent authority on hormones and the author of *Bioidentical Hormones 101*, discusses the practice of medical ghostwriting, and he had this to say in response to a woman who was told by her doctor that there is no difference between bioidentical and synthetic hormones:

I explained that her doctor reads medical journals containing ghost-written articles from the synthetic hormone makers, Wyeth and Pfizer. "Ghostwritten" is a term which means the real author is not the doctor listed at the top of the article. The two companies, Design-Write and PharmWrite provide the medical writers for hire, with instructions to downplay the adverse effects of synthetic hormones, and raise doubts about bioidentical hormones. Medical ghostwriting is marketing, rather than science. As such, it is a form of plagiarism, scientific misconduct and fraud. The invited "author" is usually an academic professor in a university medical center serving as opinion leader who lends his name to the article. [4]

In the course of my research I have found the subject of real versus synthetic (altered) progesterone shrouded in secrecy. When a front-page article appeared in the *Wall Street Journal*, my colleagues and I thought that the American Medical Association and the North American Menopause Society, two bastions of traditional medicine, would finally recognize the validity of the bioidentical hormone replacement therapy discourse. This has not happened. In the astounding article, "The Truth about Hormone Therapy," the authors discuss the ramifications of drug-sponsored approaches to managing women's health care. "Yet hormone-replacement therapy has become a textbook example of how special interests, a confused medical establishment, and opportunists can combine to complicate the issue and deny patients access to safe and effective treatments."[5]

A major study at the Oregon Regional Primate Research Center, published in *Science News* in March of 1997, called synthetic progestins "potentially dangerous" to the heart.[6] This is a critical issue, as these progestins are the basis for most of the pharmaceutical hormones given to women, from young to older today. They include birth control pills, fertility drugs, and traditional hormone replacement therapy. Additionally, according to Kent Holtorf, MD, synthetic progestins may also increase the conversion of weaker endogenous estrogens into more potent estrogens,[7] potentially contributing to their carcinogenic effects, which are not apparent with bioidentical progesterone. Bioidentical progesterone seems to have the opposite effect, altering the more toxic estrogens so that they are more benign in the body. This is most likely due to the way the molecules are accepted at the receptor sites. In his groundbreaking—now classic—work on progesterone, *What Your Doc-*

tor May Not Tell You about Menopause, John Lee states that the distinction between natural substances made at compounding pharmacies and the "one-size-fits-all" drugs of regular pharmacies is that the compounded molecule is an exact mimic of what the body produces. It does not matter that it is actually a ten-step laboratory process to get to that molecule—what matters is that it is identical to the missing substance and thus can be used to recreate balance.

Traditionally trained gynecologists have long told aging women that they did not need progesterone, especially if they had had a hysterectomy and no longer had a uterus. This is because the medical purpose of progestin use is to mediate the effects of excess estrogen on the endometrial strip of the uterus. If a woman does not have a uterus there would be no potential for a thickening endometrium, and presumably no endometrial estrogen for the progesterone to balance. But progesterone's importance for women as both a protective molecule against many cancers and as a mood stabilizer is crucial. Its value lies in its ability to replenish that which is lost through the aging process and to reverse oxidative stress, the "rusting" of aging.

Many women have had hysterectomies and may have benefited from progesterone. This is so unfair to women! All women do better emotionally when their hormones are balanced, and for those vulnerable to anxiety, progesterone is crucial.

According to Dr. Uzzi Reiss, premenopausal removal of the uterus is not a ticket to menopause, yet he claims many studies show that estrogen production frequently decreases after surgery even if ovaries are intact.[8] Eventually signs of hormone deficiency may develop, though not as often in the acute way it does when a woman has had her ovaries removed (oophorectomy) as well.

Our research on bioidentical progesterone began at The Aspen Clinic for Preventive and Environmental Medicine with Harold Whitcomb, MD, who clearly recognized that many of the women he saw needed help with hormone issues, but he was not happy with most of the available pharmaceutical options.

Even before the confusion of the Women's Health Initiative (WHI) Study became known, we saw many women approaching or in menopause. Many of these women were noncompliant in taking their hormones because they hated how they felt on synthetic progestin. Often they felt bloated from water retention, yet still had significant effects of low estrogen. They repeatedly reported symptoms of brain fog and depression. Yet it was considered unsafe to use estrogen without some form of "progestin."

I was working with Dr. Whitcomb at this time, and we started studying the clinical aspects of natural hormones with women who were eager to try them. Then I expanded this into molecular and clinical research.

Many women responded beautifully to the calming effect of progesterone. This correlated with the findings of physicians such as John Lee and Christiane Northrup. The original medical investigation of progesterone as a therapeutic agent for PMS and anxiety had started years earlier in England with Dr. Katharina Dalton. While this work was a great start, it ignored the critical need for primary estrogen in conjunction with progesterone for many women.

Anxiety and irritability often plague women as they enter perimenopause. Many women have been helped by progesterone, yet doctors who prescribe estrogen for their patients most often ignore the immense biological and emotional protection progesterone confers. Our clinical studies have shown that a deficiency of progesterone is clearly implicated as a primary factor in midlife anxiety. Midlife anxiety is generally more extreme during the latter two weeks of the menstrual cycle in younger middle-aged women, who are still having periods. But we maintain that a lifetime of progesterone is vitally important, as anxiety is one of the biggest mental health issues of our time for people of all ages.

Estrogen also has an impact on anxiety, but we have found primary estradiol more helpful for depression and for accessing more progesterone receptors. According to Dr. Jeffrey Dach, "Estrogen receptors have been found in the brain, and estrogen increases the expression of an enzyme in the brain called tryptophan hydroxylase-2 (TPH2). This enzyme's job is to convert tryptophan to serotonin, an important neurotransmitter responsible for anti-anxiety and calming effect in the brain."[9] While estradiol does help set up the matrix for mood balancing, progesterone is still the key here.

In addition to my work with hormones, I have also studied the GABA (gamma-aminobutyric acid) receptors and how GABA inhibits the overfiring of the amygdala (the part of the brain that controls anxiety). If there is enough GABA present along with a crucial breakdown product of progesterone, the result is a wonderful feeling of calmness.

GABA is the most abundant amino acid in the nervous system, and it is unique in that it is both an amino acid and neurotransmitter. People deficient in GABA are generally more vulnerable to anxiety and panic disorders.

Our data indicate that in anxiety-prone women at perimenopause, there is often too much estrogen to be mediated by the body's available progesterone. When neuroinhibitory amino acids are used in conjunction with pharmaceutical-grade, natural progesterone, women thrive and report a sense of greatly increased calmness, even during the normally difficult premenstrual phase, which is the one to two weeks prior to a woman getting her period. This is the time when most women vulnerable to anxiety report feeling the worst.

It is perfectly fine for a woman with strong PMS symptoms, such as irritability and cramping, to continue the use of progesterone into the first day or two of her period as the biological urge to menstruate will make it happen anyway. The use of progesterone will not stop it.

Progestins are synthetic progesterones, and in my clinical practice I have only used bioidentical progesterone. The progesterone we use is made at a reputable compounding pharmacy to our specifications. It works completely differently on mood issues than progestins (typically known as Provera®, but there are others). It is worth repeating this so women understand that their best interest may not be the same as that of the company making the product she is taking, and most of the medical literature in which progestins are discussed use the words *progestin* and *progesterone* interchangeably, even though they are completely distinct molecules. Dr. Jeffrey Dach has said: "This type of error permeates the hormone literature, and you would need to write computer software to run through Medline and correct it all."

In a study at the Oregon Regional Primate Research Center, researchers removed the ovaries from rhesus monkeys to simulate menopause. Eighteen monkeys received natural progesterone, and six received medroxyprogesterone acetate (MPA), the most widely prescribed synthetic pharmaceutical progestin for postmenopausal women in the United States. Four weeks later researchers injected the monkeys with two chemicals released by blood platelets to simulate a heart attack. In the monkeys receiving the MPA and the estrogen, this caused an unrelenting constriction in the coronary artery, thus cutting all blood flow. Monkeys treated with estrogen alone, or in combination with natural progesterone, recovered quickly without drug treatment. Drugs were administered to the stricken monkeys in time, and they did recover. According to veterinarian Kent Hermsmeyer, the coauthor of two of the studies, the results were surprising: "MPA is really a dangerous drug."[10]

In another study, called the PEPI Trial (Postmenopausal Estrogen/Progesterone Interventions), it was reported that the cardio-protective effects of estrogen plus natural, micronized progesterone were similar to unopposed estrogen alone, without the implied threat of the dangers of unopposed estrogen in terms of cancer. The women given estrogen plus the MPA suggested a negative impact on HDL levels. The high-density lipoproteins are a factor in reducing postmenopausal cardiovascular deaths.

The conclusion of this research was that "Medroxyprogesterone acetate (MPA— a synthetic progestin) interferes with ovarian steroid protection against coronary vasospasm (cardiospasms)."[11] The implications of those data are far reaching because MPA is used in oral contraceptives as well as in standard hormone replacement. Recent reports from the World Health Organization Collaborative Study of Cardiovascular Disease and Steroid Hormone Contraception have requested the critical need for research to explain the increase in unexpected death or venous thromboembolism in women taking oral contraceptives. The WHO data notably included idiopathic cardiovascular deaths that correlated with specific synthetic progestins. *The study suggested that using progestin as the only means of birth control needs further study.*[12] Further it is our conjecture, based on the emerging biochemical data, that *all* synthetic progestins are suspect with regard to ongoing interference of proper blood vessel dilation. Additionally, in birth control pills comprised of synthetic progestins, the synthetic progestins block receptor sites for progesterone, creating actions different from real progesterone; this in turn causes new molecules to be metabolized that are difficult for the body to excrete. This is responsible for some of the side effects seen with progestins.

ANXIETY: A LONG JOURNEY

Amy's Story

In high school, Amy struggled with extreme premenstrual syndrome, which caused severe, painful cramps, combined with powerful feelings of anxiety and obsessive/compulsive thinking. This left her feeling as if her head were disconnected from her body. At times, she felt as if she was drowning in her emotional world. During her twenties, therapy helped, but it was the later combination of biochemical support *and* talking about her feelings that allowed her to see life more clearly.

Amy also had a curvy body, typical of women who tend toward estrogen dominance in their younger years (i.e., she had far more estrogen relative to progesterone). Many women at midlife and younger have serious deficits of progesterone that impact everything from irregular cycles to mood issues, leading to symptoms such as irritability, anxiety, and an overt sharpness of the tongue. She was also quite heavy and used food as her major source of comfort.

Amy responded well to bioidentical progesterone and 400 mg per day of GABA in a blend with other nutrients and herbs to potentiate its therapeutic effects (100 mg of magnesium, 100 mg of glycine, 10 mg of vitamin B6, 140 mg of glutamine, 150 mg of passion flower herb powder, and 150 mg of primula veris officinalis herb powder).

This is a combination we use frequently called Anxiety Control®.

The combination of GABA and bioidentical progesterone helped Amy immensely. She loved being bathed in a sea of calmness—a feeling that she had unconsciously craved her entire life. Interestingly, as she became calmer she learned some of the deeper reasons for her food cravings. The book *Addiction to Perfection: The Still Unravished Bride* by Marion Woodman changed her sense of self, and her destiny.

My colleagues and I maintain that many girls with eating disorders are indeed seeking perfection—in disappearing. How can a culture assume that by valuing women for shrinking, those women could feel strong and visible and empowered? Women have to take this power out of the hands of the patriarchal thinking that led it there—including some of the worst thinking found in women. The obsessive need to achieve, without any regard to the journey itself, leaves our souls stunted and our children twisted.[13]

THE DAYS OF TRANSITION: PERIMENOPAUSE

We are seeing increasing numbers of younger women with significant mood issues. Many of these started in high school. We see a direct connection to body type and mood issues that I elaborate on in another chapter on mothers and daughters. We have seen many women in their forties who are simply not thriving. Most of these women have been in a gradual progesterone decline for many years, but often they were too busy working, and working out, to pay much attention to their increasing irritability and their lack of sustained emotional and physical well-being for any period of time. When catastrophic early midlife crisis hits they are forced to pay attention.

Abby's Story

Abby was fifty years old, but she would tell anyone who was listening that she was forty-three. She was obsessed with eating organically and yet was always smoking pot, even though she told her friends that "she would never do anything invasive." She went to Hot Yoga daily as well as pilates and her spinning class, and she always appeared to be doing something to "get better." Despite all her efforts, Abby was chronically unhappy. This is because all of her self-help activity and efforts at "getting better" were missing the crucial component, as they were all outer directed. Her innate sense of self was that she was never good enough.

Biochemically Abby had a lot of imbalances. She was tall and fairly flat chested, with a medium build. When we see this body type, we initially assume that a woman is somewhat deficient in estrogen, as estrogen is the hormone responsible for the development of curvy bodies in teenage girls. When developing girls do not have enough estrogen relative to progesterone, their periods tend to be delayed, and they grow taller, without getting curvy. In our clinical practice, we have found that often, small-breasted, tallish women tend more toward flatness and silent rage, and less toward anxiety. This is the result of being progesterone dominant. These observational assessments developed from years of collecting lab data and from observing women generally help us with our initial assessment, although they are not etched in stone.

Abby had not slept without prescription drugs for about thirteen years, since perimenopause began (this was the point when her progesterone levels began to decline). After reading a book about menopause, she demanded birth control pills from her gynecologist for her early menopausal symptoms. This was the right idea, but the wrong prescription: the pill is meant for birth control, and it is not a beneficial drug for midlife women. Additionally, the pill is composed of a progestin, which is never a good choice for women. Instead she needed estrogen, and she would also have greatly benefited from progesterone to balance that out, which would have helped to curb her acute rage and lashing out.

When Abby came to us, we treated her with a compounded cream containing estrogen and progesterone, with a higher-than-normal dose of progesterone at night to help her get off the sleeping pills, and additional progesterone if she started to feel aggressive in the late afternoon (which was her usual time for doing so).

In our practice, as I've mentioned before, we prefer transdermal creams for hormone application, because these most closely mimic the body's own metabolic patterns. However, sometimes oral use is needed as with excessive breakthrough bleeding or insomnia, though these may need to be used in more concentrated doses. We never use oral progesterone with women vulnerable to depression, as this can worsen symptoms due to upper gastrointestinal (GI) metabolites, although occasionally it can be used for anxiety-prone women at night.

Based on my original research investigating metabolites (breakdown products) of oral progesterone, some of these can make vulnerable women very sleepy—before they get calm. This is because after being orally ingested, in any form, either swallowed as capsules or sublingual lozenges, the digestive process starts. It is in the upper GI that these molecules form. The most notable of these is a first cousin of phenobarbital, which is a potent antipsychotic drug, even in minute amounts.

In Abby's case, the hormone therapy helped her immensely. She became a lot calmer, and her husband reported that she was less aggressive and easier to live with. She was able to stop taking sleeping pills. However, her constant struggle to do more—to look younger and feel more beautiful on the outside—was not something that we could help with. It is important to note that hormone therapy is not a panacea for everything. As wonderful as hormone therapy is, we could not give her a stronger sense of self-worth—for that she needed to go deeper with therapy.

Beryl's Story

Beryl finally got married when she was thirty-nine, and she conceived the following year, following many years of hormonal irregularities. This is not young for a first pregnancy. In her late thirties, she was put on fertility drugs that made her nervous system (already vulnerable to anxiety) develop serious problems in that area. But she was determined to have a baby. Had she been paying attention, she might well have noticed that there were two people involved in the relationship, both in and out of bed. She might then have seen her new husband's eyes glaze over when the word *pregnancy* was mentioned. He did not really want a child, at age fifty-eight; he already had raised two children from an earlier marriage. His need to feel younger and hers to have a husband merged at a place that did not meet either of their real needs.

Once pregnant, Beryl had terrible morning sickness—she had hyperemesis, the severe nausea from pregnancy in which eating is impossible. For the entire second month, she had to be fed intravenously, as she could not eat at all.

Many women today are misinformed about the lifelong importance of real progesterone, especially for anxiety-prone women, but really for all women. Dr. Katharina Dalton, a pioneer in the use of real progesterone, has said that during pregnancy a woman's progesterone level surges to forty times the woman's normal amount. Many women report an increased sense of calmness and well-being such as they have never known before. Dr. Dalton explained that morning sickness is a sign that there has not been enough progesterone produced by the ovaries for a long time and that the placenta is not yet secreting sufficient progesterone.[14]

According to Dr. Alan Beer of the Chicago Medical School, progesterone is necessary for the safe maintenance of all pregnancies. The children of women who use additional progesterone during early pregnancy tend to be intellectually advanced, without much ADD or ADHD.[15]

Beryl finally consulted with a hormone doctor who specialized in bioidentical hormones and worked with difficult pregnancies. He started her on high doses of transdermal cream progesterone, staggering four 100 mg doses throughout the day, and 800 mg at night. Finally the nausea lifted at the start of the second week of the third month—often a difficult month for some expectant moms; she started to feel less acute nausea after three days on this regimen. Her doctor reduced the doses after the third month but kept her on some supplemental progesterone for the second trimester.

She had a healthy, laughing baby boy who was unusually calm! Becoming a mother felt very natural for Beryl—for about twenty-four hours she was euphoric. Then, her extremely elevated hormone levels plummeted—fertility drugs prior to pregnancy as well as supplemental progesterone had elevated her progesterone levels during the second trimester. Additionally, her progesterone had soared to forty times its normal baseline during the third trimester, which is normal.

At birth, the placenta comes away from the womb, and according to Katharina Dalton, the "high level of progesterone drops to nearly zero, within 24 hours."[16]

The result of this is mood swings often with an intensity not seen since early PMS. Usually these are cyclic spells of crying, great feelings of uncertainty, as well as feelings of being unprepared for motherhood. In about 10 percent of women this condition is severe and is called postpartum depression; this is what happened with Beryl. The symptoms are usually evocative of earlier symptoms of anxiety—but with huge roller coasters: high and low emotions, extreme crying, irritability, and confusion, bordering sometimes on delusional thinking, all symptoms connected to an extreme progesterone deficiency. Symptoms of postpartum depression differ significantly from those of "clinical" or "normal" depression, according to Dr. Dalton. For example, women with depression typically have difficulty sleeping, while women with postnatal depression usually have a yearning for sleep and can't seem to get enough of it. (Obviously, some of that yearning may result from the sleep deprivation that often accompanies a newborn baby, but not to the extent that it occurs with depression.) Other differences with postnatal depression typically include weight gain (instead of weight loss) and generally feeling best in the morning (while morning is usually when women with depression feel their worst).[17]

Beryl was fortunate in that her doctor recognized what was happening quickly and saw how extreme her anxiety and feelings of dissociation were. He got her back on her early pregnancy dosing of progesterone for several weeks, then a reduced protocol, long term. Progesterone also aids in lactation, so she was able to stay on it while nursing. When she stopped nursing and her periods eventually returned, she went on a normal dose for PMS for a woman in her late thirties: 100 mg two to three times per day for the two weeks of PMS, then stopping for the duration of her period. She became calm and rational; she also had to face up to the fact that her husband had not wanted a child and was not very invested. She was for the most part a single mom, with an older, detached husband. Sad, but true. He simply had little interest. Beryl doted on her son, but she also started to develop her Self. With the goal of having a child complete, she realized she wanted more than being a mother and a wife to a remote man. She found that with newfound emotional stability due largely to hormone balancing, she was able to concentrate more than she had when she was younger, so she started taking classes and exploring new possibilities for herself.

Joanna's Story: Severe Premenstrual Syndrome/Premenstrual Dysphoric Disorder (PMS/PMDD)

This syndrome is defined as extreme depression during PMS. Joanna had a history of emotional volatility—with periods of extreme sadness in the week before her period. PMS/PMDD is a combination of symptoms articulating more severe premenstrual symptoms. Dr. Katharina Dalton, who pioneered the treatment of PMS over forty years ago, reports that approximately half of all women's suicide attempts are made during the four days just prior to menstruation,[18] when both estrogen and then progesterone fall, or during the first four days of menstruation, after hormone levels plummet and then are still at their lowest.

Niacin hexaniacinate is a supplement that can be very useful for people who are obsessing. This combination of niacin and inositol often will produce a deep reduction in obsessive thought patterns. Inositol is a safe, water-soluble vitamin that has been shown to be an effective treatment for obsessive-compulsive disorder (OCD), while niacin down regulates adrenalin, rendering it less menacing to women prone to fight or flight metabolisms.[19] In those under the now broad "schizophrenia affective umbrella" who may perhaps be vulnerable to dissociative behavior, niacin is the critical molecule that inhibits adrenalin from becoming the fully oxidized version that is adrenochrome, dominant in full-blown schizophrenia.[20] These nutrients, combined with progesterone, allowed Joanna to feel the beginning of control in her thoughts and feelings.

PROGESTERONE: A SECONDARY HORMONE

By now, you should have a basic understanding of the importance of bioidentical progesterone and how it differs from progestins, as well as an appreciation for why progesterone is important for women of all ages. While progesterone is of great importance to a woman's health and moods, it is important to recognize that it is a secondary female hormone. Estrogen must be present in sufficient quantity in order to be properly "mediated" by progesterone. Women who use progesterone alone as an anxyolitic (anxiety reducer) can become more prone to depression, particularly if they are already vulnerable to it. The mood-elevating quality of estradiol is critical for these women. For women who are taking progesterone, the critical thing to know is that synthetic progestins are NOT the same as bioidentical progesterone.

The following excerpt from a recent article that I was quoted in offers a concise summary of these differences:[21]

> The progesterone hormone and its synthetic analog, known collectively as progestins, are not the same molecular structure and, therefore, do not behave the same way in the body. Progestins were developed because of a mistaken belief that bioidentical progesterone (i.e., progesterone that is biologically identical to that produced by the human body) could not be easily administered as an oral drug. Progestins are the "basis of all contraceptive pills and gave rise to a multibillion-dollar industry," according to Dr. Dalton. When progestins were first developed researchers and practitioners believed that they were true progesterone substitutes. We now know that they have significant differences, including:
>
> - Progesterone is essential for maintaining pregnancy, while the use of progestins during pregnancy is associated with fetal abnormalities.
> - Progesterone lowers blood pressure and progestins raise it.

- Progesterone is converted by the adrenal glands into all the stress hormones, while progestins are not.
- Progesterone promotes calmness and progestins do not.
- Progesterone relieves water and sodium retention, whereas progestins attract and hold water. According to Dr. Phyllis Bronson, this primary difference explains why so many women on the Pill and other conventional progestin based hormones are prone to edema (water retention), which can result in "brain fog" or feeling bloated.

The bottom line for women to know is: *synthetic progestins are NOT the same as bioidentical progesterone, and natural progesterone **must** be used in conjunction with estrogen.*

3

MOOD CHEMISTRY

Everything that irritates us about others can lead us to an understanding of ourselves.

—Carl Jung

Every female life is unique, yet there are passages through which all
women pass that have universal aspects. This does not mean that every
woman will struggle with menopausal anxiety or depression any more
than it means that every woman has postpartum depression. The wom-
en who seek our help are actively seeking it because they do not feel
right, and they recognize that the change in their mood occurred at a
time of significant hormonal change.

Not all mood changes are hormonally linked, nor do most require
pharmaceutical drugs, although some may, and these need to be evalu-
ated properly; that is not the focus of this book. The important thing to
recognize is that sometimes the normal passages of midlife and beyond
may be enormously difficult for many people, both male and female.
One has to be able to say that it is not all right to feel this way. The
moods of women are hardly a straight and narrow path; women who
struggle with mood issues may often do well for a while, and then spiral
downward, sometimes after a long while, if there is a major biochemical
or emotional trigger. Other women may sail through. But in our experience, the years of menopausal transition are rocky for too many women
to call it coincidence, and those that consciously recognize that things
are changing on many fronts are less likely to be sandbagged by their
own lives.

Many women I have seen in my clinical work over the past twenty-five years struggle with ruminative thoughts, obsessive thinking, and anxiety. I have done significant research with hormones as well as the GABA receptors[1] and know how to work with other options besides more and more drugs. In this chapter, I discuss some of the most commonly used mood drugs and their mechanism of action if known, as well as the major side effects that are seen. I then talk about different mood disorders and show how we are able to work with them in a more natural way.

"BIG PHARMA" AND PSYCHOTROPIC DRUGS

The pharmaceutical industry dominates medicine today. There is often a flavor in drug prescribing, which falls way short of excellence in medicine. Until recently, doctors have been paid in many different ways to promote certain drugs, and although regulatory controls have tightened, this is a culture that is slow to change. In her book *The Truth about the Drug Companies: How They Deceive Us and What to Do about It*, Marcia Angell, the former editor of the prestigious *New England Journal of Medicine*, writes about payoffs to doctors who prescribe mood-altering drugs, stating that the former dean of the Department of Psychiatry at Brown University received substantial payoffs to push antipsychotic medications for teens—medications that are now considered to be dangerous for this population.[2,3]

There is a growing concern about the development of many of the new psychotropic drugs by pharmaceutical companies. When a company researcher creates a mood-altering drug, he is given instructions based on the current area and direction of his company. This applies to employees working at companies, and also other researchers who might be given corporate grants. This is not free and unregulated scientific research. With the goal of a product in mind, this is research and development rather than scientific research.

Unlike other areas of medicine, where a doctor can get physical confirmation of a disease (such as a blood test), most psychological disorders are subjectively diagnosed based on behavior. The *Diagnostic and Statistical Manual of Mental Disorders (DSM)* is published by the American Psychiatric Association and provides diagnostic criteria for mood disorders. It is used in the United States and in varying degrees around the world by clinicians, researchers, psychiatric drug-regulation agencies, health insurance companies, pharmaceutical companies, and policymakers. Currently, many doctors use it as a primary diagnostic tool, though often the criteria overlap.[4] As a result, many people are taking psychotropic drugs, even though they may not need them. More questions arise in this area of medicine than any other, except cancer treatment.

BENZODIAZEPINES

In traditional (Western) medicine, the most common medications used to treat anxiety are the benzodiazepine class of drugs. These include Valium® and all its descendants, such as Xanax® (Alprazolam), as well as calcium channel blockers. Additionally, other drugs are used to treat both insomnia and anxiety. Interestingly, although benzodiazepines are probably the least understood and most abused class of mood-altering drugs, they are also the biggest-selling drugs in the world.

Benzodiazepine drugs are extremely effective at dulling sensory response to anxiety and can be quite useful. However, they are also highly addictive and have many side effects, such as fatigue and flatness of mood, which can induce feelings of depression in vulnerable women. According to Dr. Peter Breggin, "Benzodiazepines or tranquilizers can produce a wide variety of abnormal mental responses and hazardous behavioral abnormality, including rebound anxiety and insomnia, mania and other forms of psychosis, paranoia, violence, antisocial acts, depression, and suicide."[5]

SEROTONIN AND THE DEVELOPMENT OF SSRI THEORY

Selective serotonin reuptake inhibitor (SSRI) drugs are another classic example of how pharmaceutical companies influenced drug development. When these drugs were being developed, the drive to find drugs that allowed serotonin to remain in circulation superseded any rational concerns. Questions such as "What is the history of drugs in psychiatry?" "How successful have they been?" and "How severe have the side effects been?" were completely ignored.

The dorsal raphe nuclei are the current hot area of serotonin research. This is a moderate-sized cluster of nuclei found in the brain stem that releases serotonin to the rest of the brain. It is an important discourse in women's health as the enzyme involved is estrogen dependent. Selective serotonin reuptake inhibitor (SSRI) antidepressants are believed to act on these nuclei.[6] Serotonin is made in the brain and nervous system from tryptophan metabolism and is considered to be a major contributor to feelings of well-being and happiness. The basic premise in developing these drugs was that increasing serotonin via tryptophan pathways would counteract depression, and this makes sense; however, because amino acids are not patentable, drug companies began hunting for a different, more profitable way. Thus, the invention of serotonergic reuptake drugs (SSRIs), which have garnered extensive positive (*Listening to Prozac*)[7] and negative (*Talking Back to Prozac*)[8] acclaim.

In his book, *Talking Back to Prozac,* Harvard psychiatrist Peter Breggin refutes the premise that Prozac and related drugs are doing more good than harm. In his newest book, *Medication Madness*, he continues this theme and deepens his observations with a new term, *spellbinding*. His assertion is that many people taking these mood-altering drugs cannot identify how they are feeling in real-life terms, and thus they attribute all mood shifts to something other than possible side effects of the drug, even though the drug may in fact be inducing extreme reactions.[9]

Although Prozac may be beneficial for agitative depression in some cases, very little is known about its actual mechanism of action. Interestingly, in the biggest randomized studies involving SSRI drugs it was observed that the placebo effect was very high; people thought they felt better even after being given a sugar pill.

In our clientele we have seen some people helped with pervasive sadness and depression by short-term use of these medications, although numerous women we see complain of not liking how they feel, or side effects, such as extreme agitation or fatigue. I know some psychiatrists really believe in the wonder of these drugs—and they are justly called "wonder drugs," until the full picture is seen. I have seen very skilled psychopharmacological psychiatrists prescribe better drugs or combinations for people who were not doing well. If they are to be discontinued, this must be done under a doctor's supervision, and rapid withdrawal is not recommended.

The impetus is to look for the next great mind-altering drug, rather than at mechanisms of action that may be underlying the expressed need for such drugs.

Dr. Jeffrey Dach says in his wonderful book, *Bioidentical Hormones 101*:

> Hot Flashes, anxiety and panic attacks are estrogen deficiency symptoms, relieved with bioidentical estrogen. SSRI anti-depressants do not contain estrogen, and their use for estrogen deficiency is an abuse and victimization of women who suffer from estrogen deficiency. SSRI drugs should not be used to treat estrogen deficiency symptoms. [10]

In recent years it has been observed that SSRI drugs seemed to work better for agitative depression and less well for flat, sad mood. As a result, pharmaceutical "researchers" were told to come up with a molecule that targeted both dopaminergic and serotonergic receptors: this resulted in two currently used newer antidepressants. Unfortunately, people responded very differently to these two newcomers, though they are supposedly closely related. Women started having complaints about either that involved either extreme apathy, lethargy, or, contrarily, extreme agitation.

For women taking antidepressants who have major hormone deficits, we have been able to reduce or eliminate the use of drugs—with the agreement of the patient's primary physician or psychiatrist—by introducing serotonin boosters such as 5-HTP and estrogen. I have looked at the molecular spectra or "pictures" of 5-HTP and Prozac, and they are compatible molecules, so there is no glaring reason why both could not be in the system at close proximity. By having a molecular understanding, we can gradually decrease dependency on psychotropic or mood-altering drugs and bring up the level of nutrient biochemicals.

MONOAMINE OXIDASE INHIBITORS

Monoamine oxidase inhibitors (MAOI) are another older class of drugs used for depression and Parkinson's disease. These were the first antidepressants to be used, starting in the 1950s. MAOIs may interact with tyramine, a chemical found in many drugs, foods, and beverages. MAOIs relieve depression by interfering with the enzyme monoamine oxidase. Normally, this enzyme breaks down the neurotransmitters norepinephrine, serotonin, and dopamine in the brain. These are mood-elevating chemicals, and when there are higher levels of these in the brain, mood is boosted. Obviously, then, when they are broken down and there are lower levels in the brain, a person feels down. Today, these drugs are used much less frequently, because they can have dangerous side effects, such as extreme drowsiness and reduced focus that can impair judgment.

Interestingly, there was a study done at the Massachusetts Institute of Technology (MIT) correlating low levels of testosterone and primary estrogen (estradiol) with treatment-resistant depression. The study revealed that women who were vulnerable to serious depression had consistently low levels of these vital bioidentical hormones. This study also showed that monoamine oxidase is a catecholamine "scavenger" that devours the "feel good" neurotransmitters, thus confirming the mechanism of action of the MAOI drugs. However, by simply elevating the levels of these hormones, many of the women felt an increase in mood that had been missing, sometimes for years. They did not need these potent, mind-numbing drugs.[11]

OFF-LABEL DRUGS

Recently, there has been growing concern about the use of certain drugs "off label." Basically, what this means is that physicians prescribe drugs for purposes different from what they have been tested for in clinical trials. This has been a problem for the neuroleptics and other mood-altering drugs, which, even when used as prescribed, have a huge potential for side effects. Neurontin® is of major concern here. Although this drug was originally intended for the treatment of epilepsy, its use was broadened to include treatment for "random pain," such as that associated with that vaguest of midlife diagnosis, fibromyalgia.

SLEEPING PILLS

Sleep is a natural process, or it needs to be. Sleep is when we dream, and this is when we connect to our unconscious—some truly deep healing can occur, without any effort at all. Often when people are taking sleeping pills they do not dream at all.

Millions of Americans are prescribed sleeping pills to help them get a good night's rest. But according to a new study, the popular pills may significantly raise the risk of dying—even if they're not taken often. One study found that people who took eighteen sleeping pills or fewer per year had a more than 3.5 times higher risk for death than those who didn't take any sleeping pills. What's more, people taking more than 132 sleeping pills per year were at five times higher risk for death and 35 percent higher risk for cancer![12]

Why are so many addicted to these pills? What does that say about the distortive way so many live that one cannot surrender at night? This leads to many biochemical problems, including more dangerous drugs to stay awake, so that eventually it becomes a vicious cycle. Many women have told me that using a cream of natural compounded progesterone in high enough doses (often 200 mg at night, sometimes more), and often with melatonin, has been the greatest sleeping aid. There is ample enough evidence in the scientific literature now defining the potential harm of these drugs, and the medical community needs to look at how they are creating dependence on these drugs.

Of course, there are times when even potentially addictive or less-than-perfect drugs may be useful. Sleep deprivation is a terrible state, and sleeping pills fall into the far end of the bell curve here in that they can be helpful, even though they are known for significant side effects, such as transient amnesia. Our premise is simply that these drugs are overprescribed because physicians aren't aware of other, more healthful options besides what they learned in medical school, and what they are told by drug companies.

EXTREME SIDE EFFECTS OF MOOD MEDICATIONS

School Shooters and Mood Drugs

Virtually every school shooting reported in the media has portrayed the assassin as being depressed and "being treated for depression" with strong drugs. The Citizens Commission on Human Rights (CCHR), a mental health watchdog organization that first brought the violence- and suicidal-inducing side effects of antidepressants to the attention of the FDA in 1991, initially discovered this connection after the Columbine shootings.

In the wake of the shooting rampage at Virginia Tech by gunman Seung-Hui Cho, state legislators and civic and human rights activists began asking why Congress failed to investigate the link between psychiatric drugs and school violence. According to news from investigators at Virginia Tech, Cho may have taken antidepression drugs— documented by the Food and Drug Administration to cause suicidal behavior, mania, psychosis, hallucinations, hostility, and "homicidal ideation." If Seung-Hui Cho's psychiatric drug use is confirmed, it brings the total to sixty-one killed and seventy-seven wounded by psychiatric-drug-induced school shootings. I find it of interest that most of the reported school shooters were alleged to be on mood medications, or in a state of some level of transition in their medications, when these events occurred. For example, according to MedWatch, in April of 2008 New York–based Ablechild, a parent advocacy group, reported that

> eight recent school shooters were taking antidepressant medication at the time of their crimes, and most parents were unaware of this fact . . . The drugs being taken by the shooters have been documented to cause not only suicidal ideation but also mania, psychosis, hostility, hallucinations and even "homicidal behavior."[13]

There are credible people on both sides of this argument—the other interpretation, of course, is that untreated mood issues can cause extremes in behavior. However, I think these drugs are being overprescribed, overused, and have inherent dangers. Although the side effects of these drugs can be disturbing for many people, they rarely lead to sociopathic or psychotic behavior. Yet in my practice I see women and teenagers every week who are struggling with integrating these side effects into their lives. They are also struggling with mood issues in general, and that is why they have come to see me.

To be fair, who can predict how very disturbed people might have acted with no medication? Often people who are disturbed are looking first for attention, before their psychotic behavior overwhelms all other possibilities.

Anxiety

Anxiety occurs when there is too much stimulus at once, and the brain "overfires." At a biochemical level, the brain contains specific receptor sites for calming molecules, and when these receptor sites have the correct molecules bound to them, the overfiring stops. "Neuroinhibition" refers to the brain's ability to accept the action of calming molecules. GABA (gamma-aminobutyric acid) is the primary neuroinhibitory molecule in the human brain. It is the most abundant neuroinhibitory molecule in the human body, and it is unusual in that it is both an amino acid (a building block of neurotransmitters) and a neurotransmitter itself. In my clinic, I generally use pharmaceutical-grade GABA (available from certain vitamin companies listed in the appendix) to help women with anxiety. Many women have found this more effective than the mind-numbing benzodiazepine drugs that are highly addictive and often create numerous side effects.

The general view by the pharmaceutical companies is that drugs that calm work better than GABA, which is our innate calming molecule. Most of these drugs (benzodiazepines) operate by elevating GABA levels in the brain and nervous system, so why not use the actual molecule itself? We have seen numerous women recover their emotional stability by using and learning about GABA.[14]

Panic Attacks

In the diagnostic criteria panic is defined as sudden, intense fear, anxiety, or discomfort that seems to come out of nowhere, for no obvious reason.[15] In my work I have found that panic disorder erupts when one is unwilling or unable to look at deeper issues within themselves. Eventually, this repression causes feelings to erupt in ways that seem out of character. Often a person with acute anxiety feels disconnected from herself. In extreme anxiety this becomes a "panic attack," and this state of acute anxiety sends many to emergency rooms.

Although no one ever dies from panic, people feel as if they could. The racing heart, sweaty palms, and general sense of acute distress are all signals that fight or flight is necessary. But what if the cause is purely internal? How can one run away from oneself? A traditionally trained physician seeing these symptoms would most likely prescribe a benzodiazepine drug, either taken orally or even given intraveneously in emergency situations to break a panic attack.

Depression

There are various ways to define depression. Some psychologists say depression is anger turned inward. Often there is a sense of resignation about the future that permeates every aspect of one's being—the feeling that the way to happiness is lost and apparently not coming back. Sometimes depression is disguised as anger; in this case there may be a great deal of agitation and outward signs of distress. This is what we refer to as "agitative depression." Other times, one might experience a completely flat mood (flat-affect depression), with the inability to access any emotion. This is difficult to work with in serious therapy, and it is hard for the person experiencing it as well as for those they love and live with. There is clearly a biochemical component to mood, but that is not all. There is clearly a psychological aspect to mood as well, and each needs the other in order to nurture the way to wholeness.

In our work, we often see a correlation between testosterone and estrone (E1) levels. Many women who are producing more estrone (a less desirable form of estrogen) relative to estradiol (a more desirable form) also have surprisingly high testosterone levels relative to estrogen. Although these women are not overtly aggressive, their anger is often internalized and seething. While testosterone can be wonderful for women (it is the "molecule for self-esteem" for midlife women), it needs to be balanced by estrogen in the form of estradiol. If it becomes a dominant molecule, certain issues develop. These can be obvious physical issues, such as PCOS (polycystic ovary syndrome), or they can be deep internal and emotional issues, such as anger turned inward.

This can be a major root of depression and can lead to other serious problems.

Tryptophan

Disordered tryptophan metabolism is known to impact the regulation of serotonin in the brain, which can affect mood. (Remember that serotonin is a "feel good" molecule.) Most commonly, it has been used for agitative, as contrasted to flat, depression. Although the mechanism of action is not clearly understood, there is definitive clinical evidence showing that anger-fueled depression responds to tryptophan and 5-HTP.[16]

In recent years, there has been tremendous controversy about the use of trytophan. In 1989, more than 1,500 cases of Eosinophilia-Myalgia Syndrome (EMS) and thirty-seven deaths were associated with L-tryptophan use in the United States.[17] About 95 percent of all EMS cases were traced to L-tryptophan produced by a single manufacturer in Japan. In 1990, L-tryptophan was recalled in the United States, and an FDA alert went into effect, limiting the importation of all over-the-counter L-tryptophan products. After this limitation, the incidence of EMS dropped abruptly. However, although the contamination only affected a small batch of product, this valuable nutrient became hard to acquire. Under the Dietary Supplement Health and Education Act (DSHEA) of 1994, L-tryptophan is currently available and marketed as a dietary supplement.

The research on tryptophan is extensive. Very intriguing is the fact that only a small number of people relative to the numbers of people taking tryptophan from the contaminated batch got sick, and the majority were women. Most of the targeted were already compromised with immune disorders or other problems, and many were taking various combinations of drugs that may have been a contributing factor to their vulnerability. In essence, there was no causal element that made the situation utterly clear. Granted, there were contaminants, but there were also variables that showed enough statistical relevance (in medicine, greater than 2 percent) to create more questions than clear answers here.[18]

Recently, another form of tryptophan, 5-HTP, was discovered in several plant species, notably the African Griffonia plant. This has allowed tryptophan to be more widely available, and the chemical form is one step closer to the actual metabolic pathway for serotonin. The 5-HTP form appears to have a high safety threshold, although so does tryptophan, properly made. There is now ample data to correlate low levels of tryptophan and depression. [19]

Addiction

While there is currently no definitive biological interpretation of addiction, I have seen different mood disorders, all with a propensity toward addiction. Additionally, there does appear to be a familial tendency to depression and withheld anger in people who are prone to addiction. Most addiction has deep roots in the family of origin; however, it is hard to go on to healthier relationships without somehow resolving or coming to peace with old wounds, recognizing that not all "energies" or relationships can be transformed. The healthier we become the more we recognize where change is possible, and where it is not.

People who have been desperate often discover a new family in Alcoholics Anonymous (AA), and this can become the spiritual foundation of their lives. While this is admirable to a point, there is awareness in the greater psychiatric community of how attached addicts become to whatever they embrace. It is the nature of that particular pathology. Or as the exquisite Jungian writer, Linda Leonard, writes, addiction can be "the window to the soul"—if one survives the journey through. Dr. Leonard wrote the book *Witness to the Fire: Creativity & the Veil of Addiction*, exploring the depth psychology of addiction and her own journey through. This book continues to help many women.

THE MISSING LINK: THE SHADOW IN THE FEMALE PSYCHE

There are many brilliant therapists and analysts who have contributed hugely to the conversation of women's moods over the years. Some are trained as psychiatrists or PhD psychologists first, and some have other training, but all are trained in depth psychology. By including these ideas we broaden the opportunity for women to move into the descents of midlife and come to greater wholeness. At our clinic, I see the issues largely through a biochemical "filter," while some of these colleagues have other insights. We strive to balance biochemistry with the proper use of bioidentical hormones and nutrients so that women can feel safe looking at issues that have troubled them, perhaps for a lifetime.

The Jungian approach is a brilliant psychology for midlife and beyond for those willing to honor the idea that descent is a crucial part of life and will lead to ascent if one has courage and perseverance. There are certainly other helpful psychological discourses, and we use them with various cases. Here, we are looking at what is called "depth psychology" and how to integrate that with our biochemical work.

When I look at a younger woman experiencing depression, first I look at her body type, body language, emotional patterns, and the way she processes emotional cues. I often see a split in the mind/body integration. These girls are split at the neck; the body has symptoms repeatedly, seemingly disconnected to the psyche, but this is often not so. The girl must start to learn about projection of her own issues onto others and to take responsibility for her moods and emotional issues. Otherwise, chronic patterns of illness emerge in early adulthood and often linger into a midlife meltdown where they may be addressed fully, often for the first time.

There was a wonderful book by a psychologist, Mary Pipher, some years ago called *Reviving Ophelia: Saving the Lives of Adolescent Girls*, in which she describes how the "persona" of the adolescent girl can go underground in her first attempts to please boys in her teens. She assumes a false persona, and the real one may not emerge until many years later, if it does at all. I bring emotional issues back to hormones and neurotransmitters, but I introduce these books and ideas to give the reader a sense of what the integration of depth psychology and biochemical balancing can achieve.

SHORT CASES ON WOMEN'S MOODS

The moods of women do not start suddenly. The decline in progesterone begins the onset of perimenopause, and the struggle begins—often with years of chaos and anxiety—unless natural progesterone is brought into the picture. Then the decline in primary estrogen precipitates depression in many women. The following are some case studies of women we have worked with who struggled with a variety of mood issues during menopause and perimenopause. We worked with these women in a variety of ways, using bioidentical hormones whenever possible, as well as other nutrients.

Lilly

In high school, Lilly struggled with extreme PMS. Often, she experienced severe, painful cramps, combined with powerful feelings of anxiety and obsessive/compulsive thinking. This left her feeling as if her head were disconnected from her body. At times, she felt as if she were drowning in her emotional world. During her twenties therapy helped, but it was the later combination of biochemical support and talking about her underworld of feelings that allowed her to see her life more clearly.

Initially, working with me in her late twenties, Lilly responded well to GABA, and also to nutrients that help GABA access the brain. Once she began taking GABA, Lilly felt much calmer. In fact, she felt so much better that she stopped taking GABA routinely. As she approached early midlife, however, her old anxiety resurfaced, and she went back on GABA. Although this helped a little, she was older now and needed more. It was at this time that she came back in to see me.

Lilly had the curvy body typical of women who tend toward estrogen dominance in their younger years. Many women at midlife and younger have serious deficits of progesterone that impact everything from irregular cycles to mood issues: irritability, anxiety, and overt sharpness of the tongue. Most physicians do not understand the critical impact of real progesterone on the female brain. As explained earlier, most also do not recognize the difference between the synthetic progestins developed by the pharmaceutical companies and bioidentical progesterone.

In women, there is a critical relationship between hormone levels and the way that the GABA receptor works. The chloride ionic channel passes through the GABA-A receptor, and it is this channel that allows the brain to stop overfiring. The receptor responds to GABA, allowing the molecule to move into the central nervous system. This requires the presence of allopregnanolone, a metabolite (breakdown product) of progesterone. This can come from a woman's own chemistry if she has enough, or, in an anxiety-prone woman, from exogenously or topically applied progesterone. Even oral progesterone can be used at night, as it is sleep inducing. But it cannot come from synthetic mimics of progesterone, as there is no proper breakdown to the needed allopregnanolone.[20] This is one of the main reasons why progestins and bioidentical progesterone have such different effects on women's moods.[21]

We started Lilly on bioidentical progesterone and had her use it during the critical two weeks before menstruation. Progesterone and the calming nutrients changed her life. Once she started using progesterone cream, she felt its calming effects quickly.

We did not hear from her for about six years, at which time she called for a consult. Suddenly, things had changed for her; instead of feeling agitated, she was now feeling down. This had never been in her history. She was also having migraines for the first time since adolescence. She had worked previously with me, several physicians working with me, and Wally Simons, the head of Women's International Pharmacy. In a conference call, Wally told her that she needed estrogen. She replied, "Wally—don't you remember me? I am the most estrogen dominant woman you knew." This had been apparent in her blood work six and ten years earlier. Wally replied, "Not anymore you're not." Wally explained that as Lilly approached menopause, her estrogen had declined, leaving her missing that naturally occurring, "feeling good" state, which her body remembered from long ago. It is critically important for woman to realize how their hormones affect their moods and how this can dramatically change before, during, and after menopause. Not every mood change requires a drug!

The combination of progesterone and GABA can have astounding effects beyond just numbing dark feelings that threaten to overwhelm us in that it can also break the pattern of anxiety that can threaten to overtake reason. According to Eric Braverman, MD, the person with a GABA-dominant nature is more sensitive to anxiety—but anyone can be vulnerable to GABA deficiencies at times of acute stress.[22]

Healing the psyche is analogous to peeling layers of an onion; things emerge and recycle until they are cleared. While burying sensory responses can be useful temporarily, real healing can only happen when the underlying issues are resolved. Our work helps women integrate their biochemistry and mood so that the same patterns do not continue on and on.

Marilyn

Marilyn, age sixty, could hardly stay awake in our office. She had recently switched from an antidepressant for depression, which she felt had stopped working, to another designed to "target more receptors." These drugs both have two contrasting major side effects: extreme fatigue and extreme agitation known as akathisia. For a few weeks, Marilyn felt better, and then the fatigue started unsettling her at about 1:00 p.m. each day. She could not drive, could barely keep her eyes open, and simply had to take a two-hour nap every day.

We tested her hormones and found that they were all extremely low. Her physician and I recommended a compounded transdermal cream with two estrogens (E2 and E3), progesterone, and testosterone, and DHEA at doses that were considered physiologic. These are the correct doses to restore balance to a specific woman and are the best way to formulate bioidentical hormones.

Within five days she felt a renewed sense of vitality and a desire to connect with people she had avoided for a while. She felt a surge of sustained hope in place of the apathy and resignation she had been feeling.

Sharon

Sharon came to our office two years ago. She had been taking tranquilizers for years, during and following a divorce. She no longer trusted herself to go out without taking "just a half" of a low dose of alprazolam. In this manner she had been able to delude herself that she was probably not "really addicted." But she was. For many women in late perimenopause, anxiety rules the day.

Although Sharon had once been attractive, she now looked glazed, uncomfortable in her own skin, and afraid of everything. She had an unusual fear of germs and was becoming obsessive compulsive, known as OCD. She washed her hands over and over. She was afraid to touch many surfaces, including doorknobs, which made entering a room difficult. Fear ran her life. The psychiatrist first gave her an older benzodiazepine because it had helped her previously in acute situations, then switched her to another for general use, and then continued writing the prescriptions when she came in about every three months. But he never really explored her life with her. She was seeing him to get the drugs, and he did not do what was most needed: talk therapy. Women feel better when they talk because they heal in the process of life.

Sharon found progesterone to be the most astounding—when she began using it, her obsessive tendencies largely vanished. At night, if she found herself getting redundant, she used another, separate dose of progesterone and became calm, and often fell back to sleep much more easily than she used to. She has been back to see me recently, and we have been working with other nutrients such as magnesium and vitamin B_6.

JEAN

Jean, age sixty, came to see me after being referred from the International Society of Orthomolecular Medicine office in Toronto. She had been fighting depression for years and had been on all kinds of drugs. Currently she was on a protocol that was no longer working. She said the first year she did feel better—but now she did not. Often strange side effects show up after being on these drugs for a long time. For example, some people taking certain newer SSRI type drugs develop flulike symptoms.

Jean had developed migraine headaches, which are common; she was also confused and lacking in zest, and she felt unable to make decisions much of the time.

She had a positive genetic marker for breast cancer and so could not take estrogen, which is the best antidote for the brain fog, but not in this type of patient. Therefore, we were using specific nutrients to compensate for her lack of hormones. (With some cancer patients, it is safe to use testosterone and progesterone without estrogen, but an appropriate medical person must evaluate patients with any cancer history.)

To start reducing her Celexa®, Jean went to 40 mg per day. At the same time, we started giving her magnesium citrate 500 mg and HTP (hydroxytryptophan) at night, 50 mg.

In the morning, one hour away from Celexa®, she started on a favorite mixture we use called Brain Link®; this gave her a variety of appropriately dosed amino acids that were depleted from long years of psychotropic drug use. We also custom make our own blends through a

lab for those who wish to go deeper with blood/brain biochemical testing. After three weeks, she started having a sense of hope again about
her possibilities for the future.

She was able then to reinvent the way she saw herself in the world.
One of the things Jean found was that she was now able to live more in
the present, to stay mindful as meditation experts teach, so that she was
no longer hooked by regrets or so frightened of the future.

Karen

Karen, a renowned architect and a professor, had gone to a well-known
hospital with recurrent panic attacks numerous times. When she started
feeling symptoms, she would become hostile to her husband, the person she most needed to trust at these times. She would tell her husband
she was having severe menstrual cramps and go to the emergency
room. Once there she would get intravenous drugs to calm her down;
these would act as a muscle relaxant as well. Often the drug used in the
ER was Valium, which served this dual purpose. Interestingly, these
events always coincided with the onset of menstruation. Apparently, the
major drop of progesterone at that time of her cycle triggered immense
anxiety.

Finally, she came to us, at the suggestion of a friend we had treated.
She was transitioning into late perimenopause and her progesterone
had declined hugely; this is what triggered the desperate anxiety.

Karen had significant anxiety that she had been suppressing for
years; when this finally started to look for an outlet, she felt overwhelmed by the emotional intensity. The pattern had generational roots
in that her grandmother, whom she resembled, had a similar emotional
history. Her mother, however, was of a much more emotionally even,
repressive nature, and while there was deep love between all three
women (grandmother, mother, and daughter), Karen's grandmother
had far greater intuition about Karen's psyche, which often seemed "too
intense, too hot" for her mother.

For Karen, this aspect of her life—the generations—dominated
much of her thinking about herself. She had always felt so separate
from her mother, and she somehow felt it was wrong to be so anxious.
Part of her problem with anxiety was becoming clear: she had spent

many years trying to suppress intense emotion, and as a result, her psyche had become disconnected from her true feelings.

For women like Karen's mother, emotions were often confusing and treated as a shameful thing that should be hidden. This was a result of the postwar mentality into which many of the women we now see were born. At that time, there was a very British influence of a "stiff upper lip." This was pervasive, and it influenced how many women of that era learned about their emotional world—by avoiding it.

Susan

Susan, age forty-six, began drinking steadily, daily in her thirties, as did her husband. She and her husband became a lively and alcohol-fueled couple that was always "up" and fun, and as such, they were often invited to parties and events. She had been a professional woman working in fashion retail, and she loved it, until her marriage and drinking derailed her.

Her family of origin had a legacy of alcohol and other mood disorders for generations, often with men, although there was significant depression and anger in women also. In earlier days bipolar depression was labeled manic depression, and Susan could remember a grandmother being up for days, then not being able to get out of bed. She also had an aunt who was known for flying into big rages over minor issues; another aunt who became cold and withheld emotionally after drinking. These issues existed on both sides of her family.

Alcohol enhanced her husband's already angry persona—he became angrier after drinking, and more tightly controlled in general, the anger right below the surface. In contrast, drinking caused Susan to become withdrawn and depressed, exacerbating her tendency to flatness and depression. Withdrawal and silence are lethal relationship weapons in the hands of certain women. Usually doctors prescribe mood-elevating drugs for these women when often what they need is estrogen as a first attempt to balance mood. In Susan's case, first her doctor put her on one cocktail of antidepressants, then when she said the drugs made her jittery, added a benzodiazepine that brought back the old flatness. A further change was made three weeks later adding a "medication booster drug" that has never been effectively studied with all these various combinations but has been used off label, sometimes helpfully for short-term situations.

Susan's blood estrogen level was 42 pg/ml on the twentieth day of her menstrual cycle—very low. Ideally, it should be above 80 pg/ml, even in a woman who is menstruating but probably no longer ovulating. Her new gynecologist gave her birth control pills to address the low estrogen—addressing the estrogen was correct, but not with birth control pills; these made her more depressed because of the synthetic progestin and its effect on the brain. Then a girlfriend told her about our work with transdermal creams.

My medical partner examined her blood levels, and we discussed her case as she had requested. My colleague ordered a compounded cream of estradiol and estriol with a low dose of progesterone to be used in the morning, then again after dinner, along with extra progesterone at bed. As she was quite aggressive, we left testosterone and DHEA out initially.

We also measured morning cortisol levels, as most addictive people have difficult adrenal function, either underused or overused. We put her on glutamine, an important amino acid for addictive cravings, as well as chromium and B vitamins to reduce sugar cravings.

Christy

Christy was extremely agitated. Often she said her mind felt as if it was racing out of control. Last year her physician started her on Xanax®. Since then, she has needed more and more to keep anxiety at bay. When she came to see us, she was taking it three times a day and was feeling very lethargic on top of anxious. At age thirty-eight, her progesterone decline was the first sign of perimenopause. She desperately needed nutrients to feed and calm her brain and bioidentical, not synthetic, progesterone. She came to us and started our program to create calmness.

This involved proper dosing and sequence of calming nutrients and progesterone; when the neurons are properly fed, and the dendritic chemistry is regulated, the brain cannot overfire. Christy was astonished at how much better she felt once stopping this "prescribed addiction."

It is not my job to change anyone's personality. In my work, I try to help my clients become unaffected by what others do or say. This is a hard undertaking, the journey of a lifetime. Orthomolecular medicine seeks to stabilize one's moods with biogenic substances first, often followed by therapy, perhaps concurrently with medications, if in fact they are needed.

THE GENIUS OF ABRAM HOFFER

One of my great teachers has been Abram Hoffer, who was, along with Linus Pauling and Humphry Osmond, the founder of orthomolecular medicine. And indeed, Hoffer was the father of treating people with nutrients and bioidentical molecules way before reaching for strong and toxic drugs. I am absolutely astounded today at the belief younger psychiatrists put in drugs, even when the studies supporting their use are obviously flawed. In fact, the drug companies have funded many studies.

The most extraordinary experiments in mind/body medicine took place in the 1950s and 1960s in Saskatchewan, Canada. Hoffer and Osmond were looking for the molecule that makes schizophrenia occur. They saw grave similarities in the behavior of diagnosed schizophrenics and people displaying psychotic behavior on LSD and mescaline. They thought there had to be a molecule that was similar in the blood of schizophrenic patients and those in induced states on psilocybin and LSD. Dr. Hoffer was increasingly concerned about the uncontrolled use of these hallucinogens on college campuses in the United States and Canada. He felt strongly that any such use must be in a controlled environment with a medical person on hand throughout. He, his wife, Rose, Dr. Humphry Osmond, and other close colleagues started being their own test subjects, using these substances, and later, isolating the key molecule that they found to be similar among those who were diagnosed as schizophrenic.

The substance isolated in Abram Hoffer's lab by his lead chemist, Dr. Payza, was adrenochrome, the oxidized form of adrenaline. The startling outcome of this impeccably done research was that schizophrenics oxidized adrenalin into adrenochrome, and so existed in a semipsychotic state much of the time. The antidote to neutralizing adrenochrome is niacin, known as vitamin B_3. It was also found that niacin could be safely used to neutralize the toxic effects of a bad LSD experience. These were extremely tightly controlled experiments that led to astounding insight. Osmond coined the term *psychedelic*.

Dr Hoffer and I worked together on several cases: he on the deep psychosis and I on the mood balancing and hormones as indicated. During this time we saw a lovely, though strange, young woman, Clara, from Pennsylvania. She had been diagnosed for years as bipolar and treated as such. Hoffer came to believe the diagnosis was wrong and that she had been schizophrenic, not bipolar. She had episodes in which she was indeed delusional. She scored very high on the Hoffer-Osmond diagnostic test for schizophrenia; this was the series of questions the two had developed to enable proper diagnosis. [23]

Dr. John Connolly once described schizophrenia as a disease of perception combined with an inability to tell whether these changes were real or not. This young woman, Clara, age thirty-six, had seen many doctors, and the periodic weird behaviors continued. She would be fine for weeks or months, and then her family would discover that she had been sleeping with many men, looking for connection, and acting out in other ways.

One day her mother got a call that she was wandering through a museum largely naked and seemed to be conducting an imaginary orchestra. When questioned, she knew her name but said, "she belonged in another time."

In high school Clara had periods of dissociative behavior. A number of teens tell me that they have periods of feeling dissociative—meaning they feel disconnected from their surroundings and the people in them. They do not, however, act out in bizarre ways, as Clara did. This is a red flag for early adulthood schizophrenia diagnosis. Her mother was passionate about finding better help than the potent antipsychotics being given to her daughter by psychiatrists. They told her that Clara could not function otherwise. Clara also became extremely aggressive when cornered, and her first instinct was to be on the defensive, not to learn the facts.

She had misinterpreted gestures from boys and then men all her life; she always thought she was more like one of the boys—and that was the only way she knew how to relate and to be included. During adolescence she felt slighted by boys who were after the more feminine girl, but she was included because she loved team sports, watching and playing. But during her senior year she became so overwrought when "her guys" lost a basketball game that she had to be taken home. Something was clearly off. She was agitated beyond any sense of normalcy and kept going over and over the missed play, as if reliving it could change things.

Her mother was perceptive and kind, but with five kids she had not really wanted to see the warning signs in her daughter's behavior, until that night when there was no way to avoid it. As with most serious medical issues that seem overwhelming, most families who first encounter schizophrenia cannot believe what they are hearing.

Hoffer gave her high doses of niacin and started weaning her off whatever drugs he deemed were not helping her and possibly doing more harm. She was calm and alert and quite rational when she came to see me at Hoffer's suggestion. Her mother had heard about my work and was convinced there was something very off with Clara hormonally as well.

I have been working with Clara for about six years. She has done very well at times, and then there have been times of breakdown. These breaks invariably occurred when she thought she was doing really well and stopped all supplements. People with true schizophrenia cannot usually be off niacin therapy based on the adrenochrome hypothesis. Dr. Hoffer has treated tens of thousands of cases. Clara could effectively vary the dosing but generally needed quite high doses to maintain her mental equilibrium. According to Dr. Hoffer, this required 2,000 mg of niacin after each meal. Interestingly, most people have a flushing reaction, a flushing in their skin, from the vascular response of niacin. True schizophrenics do not flush easily even with high doses of niacin. When doing well she could cut down but not stop.

We also found she did well on a custom formulation of amino acids and certain antioxidants that contributed to alleviating her symptoms. These are difficult cases to treat, and rarely do these patients do well in therapy, but Hoffer's goal was to have them become functioning members of society, and indeed many have. We are not there yet with Clara, as of this writing, but unquestionably things are better.

HOW WE WORK WITH WOMEN

For women who have a tendency toward anxiety, the critical element at night is progesterone. We use cream, compounded to 200 mg/gm at night for insomnia and nocturnal anxiety. This has deep calming effects on the amygdala, one of the emotional centers of the brain. Some women need 200 to 600 mg at night, and this is very safe and much better on the next day's mood than sleeping pills, which can leave one feeling hung over, without proper REM sleep. And since not sleeping is really detrimental, sometimes these medications can be useful to break bad patterns, but they should not generally be used long term. For high nighttime anxiety we recommend GABA for many women in the form of Anxiety Control®, or for acute times, pure pharmaceutical crystalline GABA opened into water at doses of 750 mg, sipped over ten to thirty minutes.

If there is depression at night we use 5-HTP (hydroxy tryptophan), 100 to 300 mg, or pure tryptophan, 500 mg, ordered from a compounding pharmacy. We now know the role of hormones is crucial for mood regulation.

Estrogen receptors have been found in the brain, and estrogen increases the expression of an enzyme in the brain called tryptophan hydroxylase-2 (TPH2). This enzyme's job is to convert tryptophan to serotonin, an important neurotransmitter responsible for antianxiety and a calming effect in the brain.

Sometimes, for severe insomnia, some physicians I work with will use oral capsules of progesterone in 200 mg doses. This is an effective tool for insomnia and really helps some women, but the metabolites (breakdown products) are far more sleep inducing than the transdermal cream. These metabolites are first cousins of phenobarbital, which even in small doses can make women feel really drowsy. For some women this works well, while others can only tolerate cream progesterone, because those very strong breakdown products do not occur with cream use in the same way as they do with capsules, or any oral form. If this extreme drowsiness occurs we switch back to transdermal progesterone, which is the best general form, as long as it is in doses high enough to have an impact on the brain. It is important to note that the health food store variety is simply not potent enough for midlife women to have an effect on calmness. A physician who works with bioidentical hormones must prescribe this, and like most of the hormones we work with, it is made at a compounding pharmacy. These women often do well on certain B vitamins during the day, as well as magnesium citrate.

Some of the more severe mood disturbance cases, such as bipolar, cannot tolerate other B vitamins, so this must be examined as well. There is conflicting information on folic acid: while some pioneers such as Abram Hoffer think it helps certain deep mood disturbances, others think it may be a carcinogen at higher doses. The literature abounds with these kinds of seeming contradictions, but we follow the evidenced-based medicine as much as we can, built on a strong biochemical foundation. Sometimes the positive effect of a particular substance outlays the negative possibilities. As with anything in medicine, the question ought to be axiomatic: "Is the risk worth the potential gain?"

Many women tell us they wake up flat and depressed and experience "brain fog." The first thing we check in this case is primary estrogen levels: usually these E2 levels will have plummeted recently if depression is strong or has recurred. If a woman has had her blood checked in the past six months, she does not necessarily need to get bloodwork every time there are mood changes: she can adjust things slightly herself once she knows what to look for and is under a safe umbrella medically. Telling a woman she has no laboratory signs of estrogen deficiency because she is normal for a postmenopausal woman is like telling someone they have enough vitamin C because they don't have scurvy, the vitamin C deficiency disease almost unheard of today. By our criteria, estrogen deficiency is common. Postmenopausal women, who are vulnerable to hormonal-based depression, do not feel well when their primary estrogen level falls below 100 pg/ml. We also use l-tyrosine to alleviate symptoms of flat-affect depression.

If a patient wakes up "shaking with anxiety" and foreboding, we have them get up, eat a few crackers, and then sip GABA 750 in water; this will immediately feed the primary benzodiazepine receptors on the GABA-A receptor, which I have studied extensively. This stops the "overfiring" of the messages, notably in the twin region called the amygdalae that is the seat of raw emotion, and allows a "reining in" of emotional overcharge. It is extremely effective; often this is the only major supplement needed for anxiety. However, if anxiety is high for a woman in PMS, postpartum depression, or other hormonally related reasons, progesterone is the molecule of choice. This allows GABA to work more effectively. We have women use an additional 100 mg dose two to three times daily, then 200 mg at night to quiet nighttime rumination, which often accompanies insomnia.

COMING OFF OF PRESCRIPTION DRUGS SAFELY

Coming off of psychotropic prescription drugs for mood issues must be done safely and slowly and with a doctor's or pharmacist's involvement. Not everyone can be off drugs entirely, but many can be on fewer drugs with better prescribing.

Ginny, at age fifty-six, found her marriage crumbling and her job flat-lining and uninteresting, but she had put off leaving both for years. She was consumed with fear about change; she felt it would be very hard at late midlife. But change was precisely what she needed.

She was on a newer antidepressant, one that is called a mirror image of an older drug; this seemed to help some, though not much. Then after three months her doctor added another, a drug intended to enhance the effect of other first-line antidepressants. One of the key side effects for each of these drugs is akathisia, defined as excessive restlessness. Another side effect is exhaustion. She started to experience both of these symptoms, and the relief from depression was no longer present enough to warrant feeling these strong side effects. Eventually, she simply felt as if the drugs were no longer working.

The plausible reason mood drugs stop working is because they have burned up the available supply of neurotransmitters that have not been replenished with proper amino acid use. We recommend using the nutrients right along with certain drugs, cleared by someone like me, who works biochemically, and this makes sense under proper supervision. However, we have observed patients having intensified anxiety effects if adding amino acids too quickly, or at too high a dose. The vitamins and minerals are usually fine.

It is very important not to withdraw abruptly from antidepressant drugs; the drug must be reduced over several weeks and then eventually stopped. Failure to do this slowly can result in worsening of depression symptoms. Because of this, Ginny started withdrawing and took the following nutrients in between, at least an hour away from the drugs: niacin (time released, 500 mg) helps in any drug-withdrawal process and induces a sense of emotional well-being by neutralizing excess adrenaline; and L-theanine 200 mg for the restless feelings.

It is best to focus on most important nutrients, not just to take a lot of them.

It took Ginny over three months to remove these drugs from her system, and gradually she added more nutrients. Because she struggled with feeling flat, we added 500 mg of the amino acid tyrosine after she was off the drugs (stimulating amino acids such as tyrosine should not be used with SSRIs and definitely not with Abilify®, as we have found they can intensify some negative drug side effects).

DRUGS OR NOT? THE CHOICES OF MENOPAUSE

Drug advertising has influenced our thinking so very much. A favorite cartoon from the *New Yorker* some years ago shows an elderly woman saying to her doctor, "I think the dose needs adjusting: I'm not nearly as happy as the people in the ads!"

So why take the long and often more arduous road toward better psychological well-being of orthomolecular medicine, using hormones, nutrients, amino acids, and other more bioidentical elements? The reason is because the level of well-being attained the orthomolecular way is much higher and more sensitive to life and relationships.

Medications can be useful when someone is in need, but they are often mind numbing, a bandage over a wound rather than a gentle probing to go inward and look at the core issues.

Aging is hard. It is probably harder for women, though we certainly know men struggle, albeit differently. So if a woman wakes up feeling drained from a nighttime of anxiety, what can she do differently to change the course of this day? What could you have done differently the night before to help prepare for a more restful night? Various discourses come into play.

So many of our midlife clients are already taking antidepressants; the list of drugs goes on and on and speaks volumes about the pharmaceutical world's grip on the collective unconscious quest for feeling better— at almost any cost. Why not just take a pill and feel better? This is the choice that many women must make as they approach menopause.

WHAT CAN ONE DO WHEN LIFE TURNS DARK AND APPEARS HOPELESS?

How much of sadness and depression is "existential despair," and what part of it can be helped biochemically? Women need to recognize that when there is an attempt at balancing one's nerves and biochemistry, even deep, dark sorrow can be turned around and healed to the point at which life is worth living again. There is light at the end of the tunnel.

4

THE CONNECTION BETWEEN BODY TYPE AND HORMONES

When a girl enters puberty, the brain and pituitary gland release hormones that send signals to the ovaries. The ovaries begin to produce a variety of hormones, including estrogen and progesterone, which cause changes in the brain, skin, breasts, bones, muscles, and reproductive organs. Many different factors determine when menstruation begins, from body-fat levels to hormone levels.

Girls produce different levels of hormones not only within their monthly cycles but also throughout adolescence. In my years of research, I have noticed a remarkable correlation between girls with two specific body types and their mood disorders—and our work has shown that hormones are strongly connected to these correlations. I refer to the two different body types as "curvy" and "straight-up-and-down."

I first learned this from the work of Uzzi Reiss in his classic book, *Natural Hormone Balance for Women*,[1] in which he discussed the enormous differences in estrogen production between voluptuous, curvy young women and tall, thin women. His work showed that curvy women had extremely high levels of estrogen, while tall, thin women had unusually low levels. I then made the link to anxiety versus depressive tendencies, and I have confirmed these phenomena in my lab results. Uzzi Reiss was the first to state that one's hormonal needs cannot be addressed by a low-dose, fixed-dose standard. Most women are somewhere in the middle, with some falling toward the high end and some toward the low end of estrogen production.

My scientific and medical colleagues and I have collected blood samples on over one hundred young women and used them in this study. While not a huge, randomized type of study, the observations are statistically relevant and very accurate. That said, these are observations, patterns we see, but they are not absolute. Certainly there are women who fall outside our parameters, and there are some who are combinations of both. But generally, we have seen that if a young girl is emotionally flat and depressive and there is no obvious other reason, she is usually extremely low in estrogen at ovulation. This corroborates with the laboratory tests of Elizabeth Lee Vliet, MD, who said in her book *It's My Ovaries, Stupid!* that many young women have extremely low levels of estradiol at ovulation.[2] These girls are simply not producing adequate hormones, yet they begin to feel balanced as their hormones sputter to life.

While Dr. Vliet's data is excellent, unfortunately she often uses birth control pills to correct imbalances, which we do not recommend generally because of the progestin in them. Contrary to what Vliet suggests, we have never seen any woman feel better on any progestin versus progesterone. Our data, and that of Uzzi Reiss and many others, suggest that women of all ages feel better on real progesterone, whenever a choice is available.

CURVY

Girls with voluptuous, curvy bodies are prone to "estrogen dominance" and desperately need progesterone for balance. They often begin menstruating early because there is an abundance of estrogen.

In addition, they tend to have irregular periods. (The scientific term for this is *anovulatory*, which means they are not yet regularly ovulating.) Erratic periods are problematic because little to no progesterone is being produced in the luteal phase, or the second half of the menstrual cycle. This causes the estrogen dominance, which is the main reason for the violent mood swings that can dictate curvy girls' lives when they hit puberty.

Why is progesterone so important? Progesterone is necessary throughout a woman's life for conception, during pregnancy, and from puberty through menopause.[3] It is manufactured from cholesterol in the adrenal glands and is secreted by the ovaries in the second phase of the menstrual cycle, after ovulation (the luteal phase). It interfaces with the principal calming receptor in the human body known as the GABA-A receptor. Gamma-aminobutyric acid (GABA) is an amino acid and is one of the most important molecules for helping with mood issues. GABA has an extraordinary capacity to calm the overfiring brain.[4] While its mechanism of action is not precisely known, as medical data suggest it does not readily cross the blood-brain barrier; it clearly has a major calming effect on the neurological system. I have done extensive research with GABA and have found that when there is a lack of progesterone, the GABA-A receptor does not process GABA properly. The brain and nervous system respond by overfiring, and obsessive thought patterns—and anxiety—result.[5]

When progesterone is in balance, feelings of anxiety and upset are often mitigated and lessened; when progesterone is low or missing, these feelings can be intensified. During a woman's cycle, there is a natural drop off in progesterone levels just before and during the menstruation, so feelings associated with PMS can be quite normal. When hormones are severely out of balance, however, these feelings can rage out of control.[6]

STRAIGHT-UP-AND-DOWN

Tall girls with slim hips and small breasts do not produce much estrogen *or* progesterone. The lack of estrogen is especially troublesome. It causes late or delayed menstruation (straight-up-and-down girls rarely begin menstruating before age fourteen) and is responsible for the development of long, thin bones that have less-than-normal calcification, which sometimes leads to brittleness and/or osteopenia later in life. In addition, low levels of estrogen trigger depression in many straight-up-and-down girls. While this not the case for all straight-up-and-down women, the women I've encountered in my practice who present with mood and hormone issues tend to also present these other symptoms.

Why is estrogen so important? Like progesterone, estrogen is manufactured from cholesterol. It is produced in the ovaries throughout the menstrual cycle, with the highest levels occurring just before ovulation. Estrogen is responsible, among other things, for the development of

breasts as well as the thickening of the uterus in preparation for pregnancy each month.

Estrogen is also essential for the regulation of dopamine receptors.
Dopamine is associated with the pleasure system of the brain and is
responsible for feelings of enjoyment. If the receptors are underfed and
therefore not functioning properly due to a lack of estrogen, the brain
can become incapable of feeling joy. When there is a lack of estrogen,
feelings of sadness become overwhelming, and depression manifests.

In addition, both estrogen and progesterone act as carriers for
neurotransmitters, which are chemicals responsible for the communication of neurons in the brain. Without this interplay, the developing
psyche cannot evolve properly.

A much healthier option for straight-up-and-down girls to alleviate
symptoms of depression is supplemental estrogen *and* progesterone,
the latter during the late luteal, premenstrual two-week phase *only*.
Additionally, many women of either body type benefit from additional
progesterone during the last two weeks of a menstrual cycle; it is necessary if using estrogen to protect the endometrial lining from becoming
too thick. With young women we use appropriate doses of bioidentical
hormones to regulate the immature endocrine system.

THE PSYCHE OF ATHENA

In Greek mythology we read of Athena, a daughter of Zeus. Marion
Woodman writes that the "modern-day Athena" is the girl who "sprung
full bore from her father's head" without any feminine energy present.
Her parents' marriage was in trouble before her birth, her birth ce-
mented the trouble, and the girl unconsciously grows up trying to trian-
gulate the marriage. The "modern-day Athena" is usually tall and awk-
ward in her body, not given to grace of movement or thought. Feelings
are discarded as being weak and for lesser gals.

Is there something about the girl's psychological and biological
makeup that makes her prone to such distorted interpretations? What is
wrong biochemically? In high school, this girl would have had low estrogen. Her bones would have become long and thin, the type vulnerable
to bone loss as she matures. However, this low estrogen affects far more
than bone density. It is a major factor in flat depression and an inability

to look at oneself with objectivity. What does this mean to the woman prone to this type of anger turned inward? Sometimes this manifests as a kind of domination in the way one treats other people; the emotionally "off" tall, thin girl lords it over others emotionally. Her shadows are long, physically and psychically. The subtler form of this woman has a "quiet, demure" persona, but she is fierce and cold in her energy and actions.

THE PILL

As mentioned earlier, according to Elizabeth Lee Vliet, MD, in her book *It's My Ovaries, Stupid!*,[7] many young girls attain hormonal regulation from birth control pills. Young women with curvy body types are often put on birth control pills to help regulate menstrual cycles and/or lessen the pain associated with menstrual cramps. They usually do not feel well, and in fact, they often feel worse. Straight-up-and-down girls, however, may feel a little better because at least they are getting some estrogen.

The pill can successfully accomplish the goal of preventing unwanted pregnancy because it is made of synthetic hormones that are designed to mimic pregnancy and trick the ovaries into holding onto their eggs each month. However, an unwelcome side effect is intensified mood swings and heightened anxiety. Why?

In ten years of research, we have found that these very high amounts of synthetic hormones actually *lower* a girl's level of her own available hormones, probably by blocking her receptors. I have visited with countless women who assert that their emotional troubles started or became enhanced after being on the pill. Once again, the body is producing little to no progesterone when it's supposed to—during the luteal phase, or the latter half of the menstrual cycle, because the body is receiving synthetic progestins instead. Consequently, curvy girls taking birth control pills continue to be estrogen dominant and uncontrollably moody. When these girls experience mood swings and/or anxiety, they need proper doses of *bioidentical* progesterone, which is the same molecule their bodies would produce.

In the case of straight-up-and-down girls, because they typically have low luteal-phase estrogen, they might see some improvement in their symptoms of depression if they take birth control pills. This is because the estrogen intensifies dopamine receptors, thereby allowing the brain to access its pleasure centers again, thereby lifting their type of flat depression. This is a better, safer, and more natural option than simply medicating every mood symptom.

At the same time, however, straight-up-and-down girls do *not* need the synthetic progestins found in birth control pills. It makes far more sense to give these girls bioidentical estradiol, which is the *exact* type of estrogen their bodies are supposed to be producing, in the amount they need to offset depression. We have done this with great success. We also prescribe a small dose of bioidentical progesterone to balance the estrogen, but we also instruct that it is to be administered only during the late luteal phase, when both hormones are dropping.

We live in a drug-dependent culture, and we do not know the difference between "prescribed drugs that can become habit forming" or illicit drugs that target similar receptors. Women, and parents of young women, who seek us are hunting for a less drug-dependent way of dealing with mood than is standard practice in today's Western world. Most women come to us after other options have been tried and either didn't work or created unwanted side effects.

Our approach is not for everyone, nor can we offer solutions that work for everyone. Many parents have become deeply concerned after becoming aware of the potential for suicidal thoughts resulting from a number of SSRI drugs and reading that all but Prozac have been banned for use in the United Kingdom for those under eighteen.

TRANQUILIZERS

Sometimes, doctors will prescribe tranquilizer-type drugs for girls who are experiencing panic attacks—benzodiazepine-derivative drugs that, like progesterone, interface with the principal calming receptor in the human body (the GABA-A receptor). This enhances GABA function, which in turn creates a state of calm.[8]

The calming effect of such drugs is useful in the very short term for severe episodes in overly anxious girls; however, the side effects can be devastating. The potential for addiction is incredibly high for these drugs. Plus, sleep and the ability to think clearly can be severely affected.

Again, girls who are overly anxious need proper doses of bioidentical progesterone. I have successfully weaned many girls from addictions to tranquilizer-type drugs simply by incorporating bioidentical progesterone into their supplement routine.

BIOIDENTICAL HORMONES

While certain pharmaceutical drugs are often a mixed cure/curse for many women and girls with mood issues, bioidentical hormones are, in most cases, truly an astounding solution *without side effects*. We use hormones in the safest form and way, in combination with nutrient protocols.

The type of hormones we work with for women of all ages are bioidentical hormones, which are the exact molecules found in our bodies. Bioidentical molecules are generally not used in pharmacology because they cannot be patented (a naturally occurring substance cannot be patented, and drug companies "patent" molecules in order to sell drugs). Some drugs are effective and safe; some are simply wrong.

JENNIFER: THE CURVY TEENAGER FROM HELL

Jennifer's guidance counselor called Diane, Jennifer's mother, for the third time in a single week to discuss yet another angry outburst at school. Diane was frustrated with her sixteen-year-old's increasingly volatile behavior, but she was also concerned because there was something off balance about her daughter, and she was desperate to find out what, exactly, was amiss.

"They warned me they couldn't keep her in high school if the rages continued," Jennifer's mother said when she finally brought her to see me. Jennifer was a day student at a private preparatory school and was currently in her sophomore year. "This time, they told me she had knocked over a desk. The time before, she told one of her teachers she had her head up her butt."

Things weren't any better at home. The previous day, Jennifer had crashed into the house after school, banged her books down on the front table (consequently breaking a dish), stomped to her room, slammed her door, and burst into tears. Her mother heard sobbing through the door but was not allowed to come in and talk with her.

Unfortunately, such incidents were increasingly common and, much to Diane's dismay, gaining in intensity. Diane remembers acting this way when going through puberty, but she cannot begin to remember how it was possible to feel everything so acutely (the beauty of time is that it does dim memory!).

An Anxiety-Ridden Childhood

Growing up, Jennifer was very shy. She was an anxious worrier and had irrational fears of water and bugs. For example, when she and her family went camping, she was wary of bodies of water and always had to know how deep they were—was the water over her head? If so, she became anxious, even if she was nowhere near the edge of the lake, river, or pond. And her fear of insects and spiders caused many panic attacks, whether she encountered them at school, outside, in her home, or wherever else.

Jennifer was also a bit obsessive. Her father was president of an engineering office, and Jennifer's favorite thing to do while visiting his office was to hang out in the office supply room. She told me how she would hoard their "beautiful, sharp Blackwing pencils"—she actually had a collection of them. This sense of clutching permeated her adolescent life and relationships.

Her parents were also anxious and worried—about her. They took her to various doctors and a psychiatrist to try to get an explanation for her behavior. The general consensus was that there was nothing wrong with Jennifer and that her overly anxious and mildly obsessive behaviors were simply character traits.

Often when all the attention in a family gets focused on one person, it happens to be the case that other people are not doing their own emotional work, and so it is easy to deflect it all onto the "problem child."

In this case Jennifer's father—a wonderful, kind man—had become somewhat larger-than-life with his business ventures. Diane, his wife, was feeling increasingly left in the shadows, and as a result her old issues were renewing in late perimenopause as her daughter's troubles were beginning.

Puberty Hits with a Bang

At the age of thirteen, when she began menstruating, Jennifer's constant anxiety coupled with a new aggressiveness in the two weeks leading up to her period. She became paranoid about little things, and often assumed that peers were talking about her. Once, as she approached her locker at school, she noticed a group huddled together, talking. She believed they were planning to do something harmful to her. She became frightened and started screaming at them—even though they hadn't been talking about her at all.

Those who knew her said she was overly sensitive, unpredictable, and neurotic. She was labeled as an attention-seeking drama queen. In addition, she was constantly picking fights with anyone.

She tended to develop close, intense friendships, but they never lasted long due to her constant neediness and ever-changing moodiness. Emily was one such friend. Jennifer and Emily spent hours together until Emily started to feel smothered. When she discussed her feelings with Jennifer, Emily suggested they stay close as friends but include others. Jennifer became obsessed with the friendship, and instead of giving Emily the space she asked for, she did the opposite, thus killing the friendship.

In her marvelous book *Reviving Ophelia*, Mary Pipher says that girls like Jennifer go underground during adolescence, and in their attempts to please boys, they lose themselves.

When I met Jennifer for the first time at age sixteen, she was truly cut off from herself. She was a living dichotomy—on the one hand she badly wanted to do the right things, to please the father she adored and the mother she was close to. She even wanted to please her brother, who teased her mercilessly about everything, from her freckled appearance to her love of books to her shyness.

But on the other hand, Jennifer's emotional life was a roller coaster, and she felt disassociated from not only her friends and family but also parts of herself. This is a dangerous time in the life of a young female, as this disconnection can draw these girls to promiscuity and recreational drug use (see below). These bad choices and the thrills that come with them create a false sense of connection that girls like Jennifer live for.

Experimenting, Exploring

Physically, Jennifer was an arrestingly beautiful girl with vibrant, auburn hair and a lovely, fair complexion. She had an abundance of freckles that, unfortunately, she attempted to hide with too much makeup because her brother told her she should cover them up.

Jennifer was busty and full bodied, and when I met her at age sixteen, she was still adjusting to her hips and breasts and experimenting with showing them off. She sent mixed signals with her outfits, flaunting her curves with disturbingly short miniskirts while hiding her large breasts with big, baggy shirts that showed a hint of her new cleavage.

During one of Jennifer's first appointments, she confided she had ventured into the realm of recreational drugs. "I only enjoy marijuana, though," she told me. She liked marijuana because it made her feel "more connected" to her peers—something this shy girl wanted more than anything. However, those in her life said that when she was stoned, she was actually *dis*connected and out of touch when relating to peers.

Jennifer also confided that she was sexually active. She had had sex with several boys by the time I met her, even boys she didn't know, hoping they would like her (unfortunately for Jennifer, the boys never pursued a relationship with her). When I asked if she considered herself promiscuous, she said "no" and was quick to justify her actions: "Everyone else is doing it, and I think it's one way to learn about love."

Her first statement was true, as there had been a recent wake-up call at a nearby prep school, where school officials were dealing with shocking reports of rampant sexual activity among its student body.

Jennifer's second statement, "I think it's one way to learn about love," was even more disturbing to me. Aside from the obvious consequences of toying with adult issues (e.g., the possibility of getting pregnant and/or contracting an STD), the psychological damage such behavior can cause is devastating, especially for a shy girl such as Jennifer.

Help!

Jennifer's parents became increasingly bewildered at their daughter's emotionally charged world and severe mood swings. They were also worried about her acute menstrual cramps that seemed to be getting worse. So they did what all good parents do: they sought professional help.

At first, they made an appointment with a new psychiatrist—after all, the girl was acting downright crazy. The psychiatrist labeled her bipolar but, thankfully, her parents didn't agree with that diagnosis.

The family doctor was next. She suggested birth control pills to (1) regulate her periods, and (2) reduce the severity of the cramping. Jennifer's mother didn't feel comfortable with that option, either.

I was next on the list of professionals. I asked questions not only about Jennifer but Diane as well. I learned that Diane's puberty woes were hauntingly similar to Jennifer's—something very common with mothers and daughters who share the same body type. In fact, Diane's monthly turmoil subsided only after she and her husband conceived their first child.

I also asked Diane about her *current* emotional state. I learned that while she had always been prone to bouts of anxiety now and then, she was recently experiencing more frequent and more intense episodes, thereby adding to the emotionally charged, roller coaster environment at home.

Pharmaceuticals: Cures or Curses?

Diane was skeptical when both the psychiatrist and family doctor suggested Jennifer start taking drugs for her pubescent symptoms. She didn't want her daughter to travel down the same, prescription-drug-riddled road she had been traveling on since she was fifteen.

That was when Diane's menstrual cramps had become so painful that her family doctor prescribed birth control pills. While the cramps lessened in intensity, her moods worsened to the point of becoming unbearable. Her doctor suggested she stop taking the pill and instead prescribed a NSAID medicine for her pain and a benzodiazepine for her nerves. Then, when she started having a difficult time sleeping, her gynecologist prescribed sleeping pills.

And so Diane began her long, unhealthy dependency relationship with pharmaceutical mood drugs. From earlier benzodiazepine drugs to their grandchildren, she's tried, and become addicted to, several prescription medications.

Did any of the prescription medications help Diane? Yes, but only temporarily. These drugs can be helpful to get through a "rough patch" or to start the healing process. However, in most cases, they should not be used indefinitely. This is because the pharmacology often changes over time, and much of their benefit essentially becomes a placebo effect. This placebo effect has been well researched in the antidepressant, SSRI drugs.

I have advised pharmaceutical drug use when necessary with certain patients, but only for the duration needed. The goal of orthomolecular medicine is to then use the proper, biologically compatible molecule at the proper time.

WHAT WAS *REALLY* GOING ON?

After listening to their stories, I was fairly certain that both Jennifer's and Diane's hormones were *way* out of balance. We tested Jennifer at day seventeen, because this is on average when most PMS symptoms start. She had high estradiol levels of over 600 pg/ml, relative to almost nonexistent progesterone. Instead of a normally climbing luteal phase progesterone, hers was at 3.0 mg/ml. Jennifer was feeling the effects of her hormones coming to life, while Diane was feeling the effects of her hormones dwindling as her reproductive years were coming to a close (Diane had unknowingly entered perimenopause in earnest). Diane was tested on day twenty, though her periods had been so erratic it probably did not matter exactly when, as it does with younger women. Diane's estrogen was well below 130, and her progesterone was 0.5—low levels of each, but almost no progesterone relative to estrogen. Once, she would have been prone to estrogen dominance as she is large breasted, with a major anxiety history.

I also told them they were normal, as my research has shown that each and every symptom they were experiencing was typical for women and girls with curvy bodies. They were especially happy to hear that much of their misery could be helped with orthomolecular medicine and nutrient biochemistry.

In Jennifer's case, the need for supplemental progesterone to balance out her estrogen production was mandatory. And Jennifer's mother, Diane, was also estrogen dominant and needed supplemental progesterone. Remember, she, too, was nervous and anxiety prone from puberty until well into her thirties, when she became pregnant. Because the placenta produces huge amounts of progesterone during pregnancy, Diane became calm for the first time in her adult life when she was pregnant.

After pregnancy, however, progesterone levels in all women plummet again. In Diane's case, she developed severe postpartum depression that was beyond the so-called baby blues. (Postpartum depression can be delayed in some women if they breastfeed, as progesterone production drops after birth and then precipitously again after weaning.) The term *postpartum depression* is used here, even though these are the women generally vulnerable to anxiety.[9]

Now that Diane was in perimenopause, her progesterone levels were dropping yet again. This can start to happen at least ten years before menopause, and for women vulnerable to anxiety and perhaps panic attacks, the drop can be devastating. Thankfully, Diane's mood symptoms could also be greatly alleviated with supplemental progesterone.

Diane started to feel better very quickly. Within the first three weeks there was a noticeable difference in how she felt. She was deeply pleased to have some autonomy over her feelings, finally.

Her daughter, Jennifer, is still struggling, but she is so much more accessible, less anxious, and more cheerful. If she forgets to use her progesterone, PMS is very difficult, both for her and everyone around her.

NOELLE: PHYSICALLY FLAT AND EMOTIONALLY DEPRESSED

"I am embarrassed to introduce my daughter to my friends," Noelle's mother said as she began her conversation with me about her seventeen-year-old. "She wears the worst possible things she can find and hides behind long, black-dyed hair and dark eye makeup."

Adolescent girls will often hide behind lots of hair, I remember thinking. But this was about much more than hair.

"My daughter seems to have no passion for anything except to be sullen," Noelle's mother continued. "There is no more conversation at home. She avoids me except when she needs money. She thinks I'm crazy, and I just don't know how to access her anymore."

Sullen behavior is an expression of self-loathing, psychologists will tell you. But there is much more to it than that. The diagnostic criteria in traditional psychiatry often label these girls as having "flat-affect depression" and medicate them, often with antidepressant drugs and sometimes stimulants. Every single girl I have known who has presented this way fits the definition of self-dislike, sometimes with overt expressions: excessive body piercings in weird, painful places and extraordinary excessive body art.

Happy Childhood, Unhappy Adolescence

When Noelle entered my office for the first time, I greeted her warmly. "Hello, I'm Dr. Bronson. How are you?"

"I don't know, you're the doctor," she glared from behind her dark makeup and hair, full of the sadness and anger her mother had described.

Noelle was tall, thin, very pale, and wore tight-fitting clothes. There was no trace of the happy, optimistic, and playful girl her mother said she had been until puberty set in. The girl who jumped out of bed each day and greeted her family with a hearty "Good morning!" The girl who loved being outside and was always up for anything—hiking, biking, soccer, football, gardening, a game of tag. The girl who had been captain of her soccer team not because of her playing ability (she was mediocre at best) but because of her good sportsmanship.

When Noelle started going through puberty at age fourteen, her personality went through a sea of change. She no longer jumped out of bed; she had to be coerced. She opted out of all outside activities, including soccer. She withdrew from her friends and family and started spending a lot of time alone.

To those around her, Noelle's personality change was truly epic, and to Noelle, it was depressing. She, too, missed the happy kid she used to be, and she hated feeling so out of control of her emotions. She was confused about her constant sadness and this new desire to be alone, or with the wrong kinds of kids. Some of her closer soccer friends continued calling her, asking her to do things with them, but they eventually gave up because Noelle consistently declined their invitations.

Like her mom, Noelle was also embarrassed about her sullen behavior. She felt as though she *should* have been able to pull herself out of her funk, but she simply couldn't.

Slipping through the Cracks

Noelle's personality wasn't the only thing that changed once she entered puberty. Once a driven, A-honor-roll student, she stopped studying. She even lost interest in English and writing, which were her favorite subjects. Noelle's grades started to slip, and her teachers said she had become "vacant" while in class—a stark contrast to the bright student who had always participated in class discussions.

Socially, she spent less and less time with her soccer friends and more time with a crowd at school that had a reputation for using drugs. Even though she spent time with this new group, she didn't consider any of them to be her friends. She frequently went out to clubs with this new group and started taking the recreational drug Ecstasy on a regular basis.

Ecstasy is a stimulant drug that enhances feelings of pseudo love and empathy. However, people have died from using it—it can be damaging to the central nervous system, and it inhibits the body's ability to regulate temperature.

Noelle knew all of this. But she continued to take it because the stimulant-type drug made her *feel* happy, if only temporarily.

Quick "Fix"

Noelle's parents were very concerned about all these changes in their daughter, and with good reason. So, just as Jennifer's parents did, they sought professional help.

They first took her to a physician, who diagnosed her as depressed. He prescribed a drug cocktail of antidepressants approved for use in adults, although at the time, these drugs were increasingly being prescribed to teenagers. In addition, he suggested she start seeing a therapist.

Noelle's depression lifted within a few weeks of taking the medication. While she didn't return to the happy-go-lucky, prepuberty Noelle, she did engage in conversation with her parents and a couple of soccer friends more frequently, and she started paying more attention to her schoolwork.

Soon, however, she became emotionally "flat," meaning she was incapable of joy or sadness. For example, Noelle's family was planning to go on a beach vacation—Noelle loved going to the beach—but she was literally unable to get excited about having her feet touch the sand again. Noelle questioned this lack of feeling and didn't know what was worse: the agitative depression or the drug-induced flatness.

Noelle was also questioning her therapy sessions. She spent the majority of the time with her therapist talking about her childhood, which had been carefree. She didn't have any "skeletons" in her closet, but her therapist was determined to find some. When the therapist switched to the present and tried to figure out if something had happened at school or on the soccer field to make her so depressed, she just shrugged her shoulders.

Noelle could not articulate what was wrong because her brain chemistry was profoundly disturbed. I have found that this is common in teens with mood disorders. Consequently, while I believe that therapy is beneficial for many teens, I usually only advocate it after the brain-chemistry issues have been addressed because, as with Noelle, some teens are simply miserable and are unable to articulate *why*.

A few months after Noelle started taking the medication, the U.S. Food and Drug Administration issued a public health advisory stating that SSRI medications such as the one she was taking may increase a child's risk of suicide. Noelle and her parents agreed that she should stop taking the medication, and she came to me for help.

Hope

A common misconception many people have is that all teenagers have "raging hormones" and that these little chemicals are to blame for the horrible choices teens so often make, as well as the personality and behavior so many of them go through. This is not always the case.

After listening to Noelle's story, I let her know that she wasn't alone in her misery. Rather, everything she was experiencing was normal for long, lean girls whose bodies simply hadn't figured out how to make enough of *any* hormones yet. She was not swimming in a hormonal sea, like Jennifer—rather; she was stranded in a hormonal desert.

She was relieved to hear that I had helped many, many girls with her similar body type and that I could help her as well with orthomolecular medicine and nutrient biochemistry.

SSRIs

Straight-up-and-down girls like Noelle experiencing symptoms of depression are often prescribed antidepressant SSRI drugs. As described in the previous chapter, these drugs inhibit the reuptake of serotonin, a neurotransmitter in the brain that helps regulate mood, as it passes between cells. As a result of these drugs, the serotonin stays between the cells longer than it normally would, causing the receiving cell to recognize it over and over again. The resultant stimulation makes the brain think there's more serotonin present than there actually is, thereby tricking it into feeling happier.

As was the case with Noelle, some girls respond well to SSRIs, at least for a little while. Some are able to live with the common side effects, which may include emotional flatness (as Noelle experienced), nausea, dry mouth, restless sleep, and daytime drowsiness, among others. Many girls, however, are scared by the Food and Drug Administration's October 2004 public health advisory that brought to light what many in the health care industry had been learning: that the use of SSRIs increased suicidal thoughts. Then there's the fact that sometimes SSRIs often only work for a few weeks or months. These downsides leave many girls wondering, "Why bother?"

Depressed girls of any body type, with hormonal imbalances, need proper doses of bioidentical estrogen and progesterone (again, the latter in small doses and only during the late luteal phase) so that their hormone levels can be balanced. These are the same molecules their bodies are trying to make. In our clinical work, we have helped wean many girls off SSRIs by determining the proper doses of bioidentical molecules their bodies needed. And, as a caveat, depressed people need attention, often quickly. Sometimes mood medications are necessary in the short term, and I am not opposed to someone with a serious issue or mood problem using medication until they are functional, as long as their symptoms do not worsen.

According to Jeffrey Dach, it is "abuse and victimization of women" to give them mood drugs, notably SSRIs, when they are suffering symptoms of a deficiency of a hormone. [10]

Certain doctors treat girls similar to Noelle with birth control pills, and they have been helped; however, I don't recommend the use of synthetic progestins. The side effects and the potential cardiac risk is high, and our premise is to use bioidentical molecules whenever possible.

On small doses of bioidentical progesterone, Noelle thrived. I also gave her niacin for her dissociative, antisocial feelings, and tyrosine for her flat mood. Niacin is extraordinary as it helps neutralize oxidative breakdown products of adrenaline; tyrosine alerts the dopamine receptors that it is possible to feel good again.

It is well known that the body changes that girls go through during puberty are a result of rising hormone levels. What is less well known is how varied these hormonal changes can be. During the past ten years, we have consistently seen a link between body types and mood disorders in women, which is reflective of the differences in hormonal levels that lead to these body types. It is very helpful for women to recognize that their moods may be biochemically based and that they can have some control over those moods when their hormones become more balanced.

The women we see of all ages are having difficulty dealing with mood issues; that is why they have come to us. I always try to get them into talk therapy in conjunction with my work, as having a "safe place" to talk is an incredible gift. However, we have found that talk therapy alone is not sufficient if a women's hormonal system is completely unbalanced. Our work gives women a biochemical foundation so that they are able to better able to understand and have control over their fluctuating moods.

5

WEAVING THE WEB: HOW HORMONES ARE CENTRAL TO THE FEMALE PSYCHE

The psyche is mirrored in one's biology. According to Carl Jung, our symptoms tell us a story about how we are doing during the day; our dreams reflect this at night. In our work of balancing female brain chemistry and bringing things into physical alignment, the goal is to have women be both physically and mentally better able to handle their complex emotional worlds.

Women tell us many stories in our office, and they come for help with a variety of mood disorders. Our approach is to help them create a strong enough nervous system so that the critical issues can be looked into. In this chapter, I present some case studies that illustrate how balancing hormones helped individual women deal with traumatic issues in their lives.

DEALING WITH BETRAYAL

Pam was a brilliant, strong, and very attractive woman who had an extraordinary career and a marriage of great desire and mutual love and support. She was working with me for several years as she navigated menopause. In her midfifties, she started feeling in crisis with her husband—there were issues in their marriage that he was avoiding, and she felt betrayed by his lack of openness.

During this time, she was at the effect of loss—she keenly felt the event as betrayal, and she was upset about the potential loss of her marriage to the man she deeply loved. When a sudden drop in estrogen impacts the brain, depression can descend on vulnerable women and steal one's hope and sense of the future. This is the basis for resignation depression. Concurrently, the drop in progesterone can trigger feelings of intense anxiety and self-doubt.[1]

Our initial approach was to measure serum (blood) hormone levels. Women going through extreme stress will show a drop in levels of 17-beta estradiol, which is the most important bioidentical form of estrogen. Her level at her last check up three to four months prior had been a solid 150 pg/ml—a good level for her at age fifty-four. Now, the level had dropped precipitously to less than 50 picograms; this was very low for her and was contributing to her brain fog and furthering her feelings of confusion and despair. Knowing this, we were able to create some relief in biological symptoms very quickly.

The change in a woman's conversations with me within twenty-four to forty-eight hours of hormone treatment is often remarkable. Once Pam's hormones were in balance, she was able to see her relationship in a different light and make more rational choices. She was able to see that she did not have to escalate a potentially volatile situation and could avoid creating the very thing she most wanted to avoid: leaving the man she loved. She was able to deal with both the acute situation and some old, underlying issues, and in doing so, she became more aware of her ability to process emotions. Of course, many factors enter into mood changes; here I am illustrating what I look for and why certain women seek this approach.

Sudden drops in estrogen can also produce headaches, which further perpetuate the lack of well-being so needed in desperate moments. At our office we immediately started Pam on extra estrogen for short-term use, until she was strong, then she would go back to her regular dose. She was having headaches for the first time in a year, which the additional estrogen relieved greatly. Sometimes progesterone also helps headaches by increasing the access of estrogen receptors and by working as a muscle relaxer in its own right.

If a woman is supplementing with estrogen and a headache develops, it must be determined if some form of stress was obvious, preceding the headache. If so, her doctor could advise her to double the estrogen immediately and possibly repeat in four hours. Her headache will probably be gone. The mechanism is as follows: When the body is stressed, acetylcholine is released. In the presence of sufficient estrogen, acetylcholine causes blood vessels to dilate, increasing blood flow to the extremities (this is commonly known as the "fight or flight mechanism"). But in the absence of sufficient estrogen, acetylcholine actually causes blood vessels to constrict, causing a common type of menopausal headache.[2] At our clinic we usually use a separate tube of cream estradiol in 1 mg doses, available by prescription from compounding pharmacies.

The increase in estrogen produced an improvement in general mood and outlook within two hours. The headache got better, and it went away completely when we added an extra dose (100 mg) of transdermal progesterone. Progesterone helps stimulate estrogen receptors to work better; it is also a muscle relaxant and is calming, both of which help headaches.

In addition to hormone replacement therapy, we also started her on l-tyrosine for the sadness and flat affect. Studies at Harvard Medical School suggest that lack of tyrosine may result in depression and random sadness.[3] Tyrosine and estrogen can work wonderfully together to prevent such bouts. Tyrosine is not indicated if a woman is more prone to anxiety, as this amino acid can induce agitation. It is indicated for sadness and flat mood and for resignation, the sense that nothing can or will change. Adding 500 mg of l-tyrosine after breakfast and lunch helped her substantially.

The rage was strong for the first two days, then Pam connected to the sadness under that, and this was the abyss for her—she was afraid of falling in. These feelings needed time, as well as biochemical support, to heal. Somehow the psyche wants to regenerate. Jungian psychology can be immensely useful here because those willing to look can see themselves as universal archetypes, rather than literally. It is not always personal. The world of Jungian literature is rich with books to support midlife meltdowns. Some of my favorites are any books by Linda Schierse Leonard or Marion Woodman, particularly *The Wounded Woman* and *The Pregnant Virgin*, respectively. I also love *Psyche Speaks* by Russell Lockhart, *The Heroine's Journey* by Maureen Murdock, and anything by Marie-Louise von Franz; a special one is *Shadow and Evil in Fairy Tales*.

Talk therapy in general can be remarkably helpful as adjunctive therapy, especially when it is partnered with biochemical changes; without biochemical support, people tend to get stuck in telling their story, but not really changing. We often give women homework in the form of various books to read and discuss in the context of whatever mood issue is going on.

FINDING ONE'S STRENGTH AT MIDLIFE

Laurie chose a life of ease: she married a man with a substantial trust fund. However, soon after her marriage, she realized that he was an arrested adolescent. The term for this type of man is the *puer* in French, known as "Peter Pan" in American literature, the man-child who refuses to grow fully into mature adulthood. No one has ever challenged the boy/man's way of showing up in the world. He gets invited to the party not because of who he is but because he inherited money. Laurie married into this swamp of adolescence—the need to dominate and control.

Whenever they would argue, he would say he was leaving because she was angry—then he would move into a luxury hotel, leaving her and their three children behind. The last siege lasted six weeks, until he said he was ready to come home. Laurie had reached her limit, and this time she insisted that he go to therapy. A woman has to become strong enough to be willing to let go of clutching at something that is not working repeatedly in order to get to this point.

Laurie was an extremely estrogen-dominant woman, and progesterone helped her immensely by calming her negative obsessions about herself—those thoughts that said, "If I was good enough, he wouldn't act this way." She needed to understand that his actions had nothing to do with her, and this is what her calmer brain allowed her to see.

We always look at blood tests, and then our conversations are structured to obtain biochemical direction through a psychological inquiry. Laurie was still menstruating regularly, so I measured her blood on day twenty-one of a normal twenty-eight-day cycle. Her estrogen at this second postovulatory peak, in the luteal phase, showed high estrogen (450 pg/ml) for a woman of this age, and an almost nondiscernible amount of progesterone.

I treated her with just progesterone, then added testosterone after two weeks. She had come to me with repetitive negative obsessions, and within two weeks, she began to feel better about herself. At the time, she did not require any estrogen, as she was quite estrogen dominant, even at age forty-eight. In our experience, women who are estrogen dominant when they are younger often experience a precipitous drop in primary estrogen as they approach menopause, but for the time being, progesterone gave her the sense of calm that had eluded her for years, while testosterone gave her the courage to start to look at why she had married this person and had three children with him. This and talk therapy allowed her to see that it was much better to live on one's own and struggle for a while then to live in a relationship based on survival.

HORMONAL CHANGES AFTER A HYSTERECTOMY

Virginia came to me after having a hysterectomy that she later believed was unnecessary. Since the surgery, she had been having persistent symptoms of depression, rage, and sadness.

We tested her hormone levels, and her testosterone blood level was much higher than her estrogen, making her quite aggressive (in her eyes—more like a man). She was quite proud of this and felt it kept her from getting too attached to relationships the way other women did, and she considered this a sign of strength. My perception was that she was well on her way to becoming a bitter and alone old woman if she did not look underneath her superficial sense of who she was and how she operated. I worked with her gynecologist to get her on a com-pounded formula that contained E2 (estradiol), E3 (estriol), and pro-gesterone. She also used extra progesterone at night, in the form of a 200 mg cream.

She did, by her own admission, become less aggressive and more willing to listen and be receptive—clearly aspects she desperately needed to develop. But she would not go to talk therapy and look at herself deeply. Thus, the first time she got mad at me for some minor thing—she did not like my answer to her question about how her anger showed up—she stopped communicating. Ah, the deadly toxicity of silent rage.

I have not seen her in some time, which is probably okay, because I cannot make a difference with someone like this unless they congruently are in therapy. The biochemistry can only do so much. It takes real work to get under some of these very deep issues, and if a woman is looking for a quick fix, this is not the best route for them to take.

SELF-DECEPTION AND THE INFLATED SELF

I have worked with countless women over the years, and helped most of them, although there are certain types of women that I have a difficult time working with. One of these is the very busy woman with a very high view of herself, no matter what occupation or role she plays in her life or in the lives of others. "Self-inflation" is the hardest personality disorder to treat, in my experience. Narcissistic patients are unable to face their own grandiosity, thus it becomes their persona, how they manifest in the world. Often these women are prone to anorexia, or some other type of self-destructive behavior, as well as behaviors that are destructive to those around them. They may use recreational drugs, particularly marijuana, now under the guise of medical need when there is no such purpose whatsoever.

One woman, Claudette, was an expert at self-deception. She came in with all good intentions, wanting to improve. In fact, improvement was her whole deal; she went to everything in her endless quest to be better. She was "addicted to perfection," as Marion Woodman describes in her wonderful gem of a book by that same title, yet my observation was that she was cold, fearful, and brittle inside. By her own admission, she had married a man for his money, which his father had made. She did not like or respect her husband, but she also didn't want her lifestyle to change.

After a few visits with me, it was clear that hormones alone were not going to change her. She was married to her lifestyle and unwilling to do the work required to get out of the rut she was in. As much as I would have liked to help her, I had to let her find her own path.

I have another client in her early fifties who has a major need for one-upmanship, making her also very difficult to work with. In my office she would get very intent—not on getting the help she desperately needs—but on telling us how much she knows. When we tested her hormone levels, she was (not surprisingly) very low in progesterone. She needed a great deal of progesterone before she could even begin to slow down to observe these things, as she was extremely hyper in her speech and actions, yet she was afraid to use too much progesterone because she thought it would make her gain weight. She likely thought this because synthetic progestins can cause significant weight gain due to water retention. We repeatedly told her that bioidentical progesterone would not cause her to gain weight, but she would not listen to us. I finally realized after about a year that I couldn't help someone who was married to her ego. In this way, this is not about my work, it is about their life—and while the hormone progesterone can indeed slow a woman down so she could start to think . . . she has to recognize there is a problem.

I think of another woman who was a life coach. She was incredibly intense and anxious, which are the first signs of progesterone deficiency in women, and she had two teenage daughters manifesting similar emotional patterns. She had an ardent need to justify her work, how "even though she was not trained as a psychologist she had much to offer." And I was confident that she did have a lot to offer once she felt more in balance with her own life.

In high school and college, Leslie had been a nice girl, not outstanding, and she did her best to blend in. She wanted to finish college engaged, and she seemed willing to settle for anyone acceptable (wealthy). She always took the easy way out. She finished college with no real significant interest in academics, and she got engaged. They lived a pleasant life, very security oriented, and they had two children. When the oldest was in college and the younger finishing high school, her husband had an affair with someone at work. She left him and decided to become a life coach. She was determined to run a marathon the following year to show something to her obsessively athletic ex-husband.

At the time she came to me, she was feeling anxious and driven. She had probably been deficient in progesterone all her adult life, since puberty. After initial testing, I gave her a blend of amino acids formulated to be suitable to her chemistry. Once she started both hormone and amino acid treatment, she became a calmer, more balanced woman, and for the first time she started to look at her tendency to bypass real work and look for instant glory and gratification. I worked with her for a while, and I also referred her for therapy but felt she did not need it because of her life coaching. I have not seen her now in several years, but I have heard from others that she is doing well and seems to be getting her life back on track.

HORMONES FOR BREAST CANCER SURVIVORS

Ellen, a financial consultant, came to see us for help managing her sharp tongue and edgy mood swings. Even though she came to us, she felt like hormones were not for her, as she understood her moods. Before we even started to work with her, Ellen was convinced we had very little to offer, so much so that my colleague, a physician on her case, asked her, "If you already know the answers, then why do you want our input?" She refused to take hormones, and of course that is her choice; this approach is not for everyone, yet she had come to us for help. Because she wouldn't listen, we never got to explain to her that bioidentical hormones per se do not cause cancer and that proper hormonal balance can actually be a basis for resisting cancer, if the genetics are not overwhelming. A year later she was diagnosed with breast cancer.

This was an amazing process for her. Initially, she was so terrified that she immediately requested a double mastectomy, which was not at all indicated in her case. Thankfully she had a conservative, intelligent physician who persuaded her that one breast only was afflicted. She had surgery and then traditional hormone repressive treatment, and after a few initial scares, she has done well, but she has aged rapidly with the drug she is on, Arimidex®; this is widely prescribed for women after breast removal for cancer, and while it may help save some women, many feel so terrible from it they can barely function. When she came back to consult with a colleague of mine, Ellen felt old and depressed— due both to the trauma of the surgery and the postsurgical medication she was taking.

Of course, after cancer, with estrogen-positive receptors, she was not given estrogen. But a colleague of mine had been studying protocols using bioidentical progesterone and testosterone for women with depression after breast cancer. There are eminent physicians working on these issues around the world. This combination of hormones helped her moods enormously, and she began to look at her history of incessant activity. She realized that her held positions on everything were linked to why she attracted what she most feared—being like her mother, who had been a rigid and controlling woman. Three men had been interested in her before she became ill; she rejected each because they wanted more intimacy than she could tolerate. When they left her she become hysterical, and each repeat crisis left her more blaming and victimized. According to Carolyn Myss, author and medical "intuitive," women cannot be consciously creating their own reality and be victims of anyone or anything at the same time.[4] One must be ultimately responsible. Ellen found it very hard to admit to needing therapy, and yet after developing breast cancer, she started seeing a Jungian analyst in New York. Jungian therapy is beneficial for people in midlife and beyond because Jung's emphasis is based on the premise that people do not really become interesting until they volitionally—or by default—move through at least one major midlife crisis. Many people do this without waking up. For those that heed the call, life becomes incredibly meaningful and profound, new again. But the descent is very precipitous for someone as rigidly held as Ellen. She had a superlative therapist, a woman of great insight and toughness and compassion. She started awakening the mystical power of dreams in Ellen because this was the route to the locked-up psyche, so long frozen under layers of false smiles and the presumption that Ellen knew what was right for her friends, and everyone else. Ellen had been out of hormonal balance for most of her adult life, and her psyche was damaged. She had to get to a point physically where she could look at her underlying emotional issues.

After getting bioidentical progesterone for just three weeks, Ellen was able to sleep deeper and began remembering important dreams. She started to dream of a male figure who had a seemingly "nice" persona but was secretly a very nasty guy. This dark, patriarchal figure would not leave until Ellen started to see consciously that the men she was attracted to were infantile in their male development. She finally dreamed that she asked him to leave and he did. About a month later she started dreaming of a male figure who was a warrior, fighting for her. Dreams are the way the unconscious speaks at night, showing the direction one is hopefully moving toward. This was a step up; seeing a man symbolically looking out for her best interests was new territory for her, and her unconscious (dreams) were leading her into new possibilities.

OLDER WOMEN NEED THEIR HORMONES, TOO

The current idea in medicine is that women should only take hormones for five years postmenopause. However, this does not make sense to those of us working with women and depression. The medical concerns have to do with estrogen's impact on vascular function, but most of the hormonal studies have been done with synthetic hormones as mentioned earlier in this book. Our concern is that estrogen and progesterone have a huge impact on women's moods, whether they are experiencing depression or anxiety.

Progesterone, as you have now learned, is the great molecule of calm and has a magnificent role to play in the nervous systems of women of all ages. Women with great emotional balance are a joy to their families, friends, and work—often healthy women can work a lot longer—and they are at peace with themselves.

Recently, I have seen some wonderful women in their sixties and a few in their seventies. Some of these have had late midlife shakeups in very complacent prior lives that have been truly psyche shattering. Ah, an opportunity to rebuild and for a new life, perhaps.

In recent years, I have learned so much about how to help women in this slightly older group, even though I am younger than they are, because of the sorrow of losing my husband so soon. What I have come to see is that learning about how to renew one's trust in life and regain a sense that one can indeed be happy again are based on courage, resilience, and perseverance: never give in to defeat or fear or sorrow. This is a very distinct discourse from accepting something that must be accepted, such as a death. Short of that, wherever there is life, there is hope.

One woman discovered that her husband had been philandering for years—but with the same woman. There is something wrong with a man who would behave this way, such that his narcissism is so grandiose that he cannot see the damage he leaves. The woman who came to me was a very bright, accomplished one, and she thought she lived in an exciting marriage with a very ambitious, type-A guy who was known to be very cold—but with her, he seemed . . . content enough.

When the infidelity was discovered, it was worse than just feeling betrayal; it was a betrayal of an entire life of marriage. How would she survive the staggering overnight dimming of her self-esteem? She was used to having it all. Indeed, this woman had never known any hardship, and she thought she was safe and secure. She had gone from a wealthy and protective—though distant—father to a wealthy man's bed. She had worked hard and been successful in her own right. However, this marriage blinded her to her own valuable self-worth because he was such a cold man, and she thought that for him to choose her, she had risen somehow as a woman, rather than valuing herself first.

This woman came to me because she became concerned that the drugs a psychiatrist had her on felt like way too much. I worked with a local psychiatrist who weaned her off excessive medication and put her on only one medication (she had been on four); she was a walking zombie who did not want to feel anything. But that is hard to wake up from, the raw contact with remembering what happened.

Many women when going through a crisis ruminate to the point at which their minds are crowded with unwanted thoughts. Part of our work beyond balancing hormones and mood biochemistry with nutrients is to allow the woman to command the direction of her thinking. Instead of "I want the jerk back," no matter how much abuse he will heap on her again (which is what she had been doing), the return of her hormones from nothing to healthy levels helped her to see that she really didn't want to be with an abusive man, no matter how much she had invested in their former life together. Some women will hang onto the idea of a certain connection that feeds a certain set of emotional wiring that she has: Jung called this feeding a complex. Once the woman does some very deep soul searching, she can come to a new level of wholeness and never look back.

One of my favorite clients over the years has been a very elegant European woman who lived part time abroad and part time in New England. She was one of the first clients I worked with, when I was working with neurotransmitters and before I was even studying bio-identical hormones. She had an austerity and elegance about her, yet she had been overcome with a major anxiety disorder after the birth of a second child. Her family could not begin to accept that she had a biochemical tendency toward anxiety—and so they pathologized her needs as being "crazy or somehow dysfunctional." They did not see her anxiety as a medical condition at all. In fact, this thread of anxiety exists throughout her family, though unconsciously. She, however, was looking for alternatives, and she began working with me. She claims that my early work on anxiety (using just neurotransmitters) saved her life.

She suffered a great deal. When I met her she had been in and out of mental health facilities and been to many emergency rooms over several years. This was years ago, and she was then forty-eight, about five years after her second child was born. We started her on regular doses of GABA (gamma-aminobutyric acid), which is a neurotransmitter; she responded best to our pure crystalline 750 mg capsules. She needed to open these and put them in water and sip; this is the best way to take these higher doses of GABA—under 500 mg they can be swallowed.

For those with panic disorder the higher doses are recommended. I have done a great deal of original research on the GABA-A receptor and how this works. Later, in more recent times, this became integral to my hormone research.[5] At the time that Angeline first came to me we started her just on GABA, as my research with hormones had not yet begun. She thrived and was able to get off the psychotropic drugs (benzodiazepines had initially calmed her, though she had come to hate the dullness and other side effects). She had become hugely dependent; these drugs are highly habit forming. So for a number of years things worked well. Years later, she started progesterone, and this truly produced the link to deeper calmness that had been missing all her life.

Other women are more stoic in their choices. I recently went to a memorial service of a woman who was part of an older circle of friends who are all ten to twenty years older than I. I felt the sadness of her passing certainly, but also sadness at her stubbornness.

She would express fascination for what I do in my hormone research but would not consider learning about my work for herself, as it did not fit in her pictures of Western medicine of which she seemed overly fond. Most heart disease in women starts after menopause and is the biggest killer of women by far, yet the prevailing medical and media focus remains on cancer. Had this woman been taking good estrogen and some protective progesterone, she may have been able to avert the heart attack that claimed her suddenly and completely.

As women age, the tendency toward inflammation increases as the level of their good estrogen (E2) decreases. In some people, the inflammatory response is triggered inappropriately or never fully shuts off, potentially resulting in a state of chronic inflammation. Blood tests have detected low levels of inflammation in people diagnosed with a wide variety of illnesses. For example, the "silent" inflammation of cardiovascular blood vessels is now widely believed to be a key part of atherosclerosis.[6] Exactly how biochemical processes cause chronic inflammation is not yet understood, but we do know that women and older people suffer more inflammatory illnesses. "Inflammation is a particular issue for women during and after menopause," notes Marcelle Pick, a nurse practitioner at Women to Women Healthcare Center in Portland, Maine. "Somehow—and we're not sure yet how—this hormonal transition stokes the fire. Inflammation caused by hormonal imbalance could be a key reason why women suffer 75% of all auto-immune disease." Women are not aware that a chronic state of low-level inflammation can reduce their chances of aging well.[7]

A 2003 study published in the *Journal of the American College of Cardiology* suggested two possible keys to this puzzle regarding estrogen's effects on inflammation:

- the type of estrogen
- the route of administration

This study of twenty-six women, which compared the administration of two different types of estrogen, showed that oral conjugated equine estrogen pills (Premarin®) doubled CRP (C-reactive protein, an inflammatory marker in blood) levels and lowered levels of an anti-inflammatory growth factor (insulin-like growth factor-1 or IGF-1). Conversely, estradiol (Climara®) delivered via a transdermal patch did not increase markers for inflammation. "Because CRP is a powerful predictor of an adverse prognosis in otherwise healthy postmenopausal women," the authors concluded, "the route of administration may be an important consideration in minimizing the adverse effects of ET [estrogen therapy] on cardiovascular outcomes."

The woman I mentioned who had just died of "silent heart disease" had been very involved medically and knew a lot for a layperson. She had been on a major university medical review board as a layperson member. Yet her own heart disease went undetected, and she was taking a statin drug that she hated as her joints often hurt since starting it. She also talked about shortness of breath, which can be attributed to heart disease or may be a function of a deficit of CoQ10. She had taken herself off hormones after the halting of the Women's Health Initiative (although I think she needed estrogen very badly). The day that I witnessed her friends and relatives grieving, I was the only one wondering what might have been done preventively. The webs we weave over many years show up as feelings of loss and betrayal, silent inflammation, and perhaps unnecessarily untimely death.

The cycle continues—yes we all age and die, but this one seemed . . . preventable.

> Great crises often provoke hidden resources and can reveal the underlying unity of life. At critical moments in history mythic sense tries to return and indicate life's inherent capacity for renewal . . . In times of change it becomes important to have a narrative feel for life and a reverence for the unseen presence of eternity. Being alive at this time means being near the threads of existence and invited to participate in the great reweaving of the garment of life.[8]

6

SEXUALITY

For years, women have thought of their own sexuality in terms of relationships. Women have been told that sex for them is "relationship based" and that their sexual desire is a direct result of being in love. Unfortunately, for many women, things are not quite so clear in their own experience. A riveting report by Meredith Chivers, presented in *New York Times* magazine by Daniel Bergner, casts doubt on some ancient thinking in this arena. The article "What Do Women Want?" created an uproar in the field of female sexuality, as has much of Chivers's work. Notably, it was shown that sexual arousal in women may be extremely physical and may also be considerably detached from love relationships.[1]

Chivers and her colleagues have been in a hotly contested debate with the psychological orthodoxy in this somewhat subjective area of human biology. Sex has long had Freudian overtones, and every aspect has an emotional overlay. In her research, Chivers asserts that women can become aroused through observation of mildly stimulating pictures. One of her examples suggested that watching other women could stimulate women. A naked woman exercising appeared to exert a strong sexual urge in a statistically relevant number of women. Why? The question begs a look at the relationship between hormones and sexuality.

Many women come to our clinic saying they have no sexual desire and no interest in sex, even with men they deeply love. (I have not heard the same response from lesbian women, but I have not worked with as many.) For men, sexual rejection means they are no longer valued or loved. For women this lack of desire may be part of the loss of sexuality that accompanies menopause and may have nothing to do with other associations of love, and yes, even desire. However, the desire to take action is missing. Many women feel guilty at not wanting to either initiate or respond sexually. Often this can go on for some time and has ruined countless relationships. There are many visits to therapists as women frantically try to figure out the truth about their relationships. But what if part of the answer is not in the psyche? What if women are not turned on simply because they have low levels of testosterone and estrogen?

According to Barbara Sherwin of McGill University, who has studied hormones and menopause extensively, there is a time-limited period in menopause when the ovaries produce more testosterone as the production of estrogen and progesterone halts. However, this is of short duration and can be deceptive. Once they are fully postmenopausal, most women do not produce significant amounts of testosterone.[2]

Many women with no libido are low in testosterone, and because it is quite potent in small amounts, they need very little to have a sexual impact. Testosterone does not have to be applied directly to sexual organs to be stimulating; it can be applied as a cream and is absorbed into the bloodstream in the same manner as other hormones.

As mentioned earlier in this book, testosterone has a great deal to do with self-esteem as well as sexual desire. Self-esteem is a dominant issue of ongoing testosterone deficiency in many women; they are much more concerned about this than any other factor. Most likely, this is because perception impacts mood so greatly. If a woman perceives that she is more able to produce effective action, she is more likely to do so. While the act of being decisive is traditionally associated more with male health, at midlife the lack of this ability becomes a very big issue for women. Many women have told us that when this ability returns, libido follows.

We have done many blood tests over the years, and many women fall well below measurable testosterone status at less than 20 ng/dl. Most women feel best when their blood levels of bound testosterone are above 40 to 70. If testosterone levels get too high relative to the female hormones, I observe that women become aggressive rather than appropriately assertive, which is what we are aiming for.

Susan had been a very active, vital woman until menopause. Her primary physician prescribed the Vivelle® patch, a decent source of estradiol. Although her mood improved, her energy, libido, and sense of self-worth didn't change. She found herself indecisive and unable to commit to her decisions. These are all signs of testosterone deficiency.

Susan started using a small amount of testosterone cream transdermally, 1.5 mg daily, applied to the skin. After one week, she felt her sense of purpose returning; after a month her general sense of female empowerment came back.

Nancy was very happy in her relationship and had been married for twenty years. Her loss of sexual desire made her sad, but she still thought she was happily married. Her husband thought otherwise and let her go along without discussing his changing feelings. He assumed she no longer desired him, not realizing that she simply had no desire. Feeling rejected, he started having a flirtation with someone at work— someone he would not have been vulnerable to in the past. When Nancy observed them talking at a party she was able to intervene before anything developed, but her marriage was hanging on a cliff. Her husband told her that he thought she couldn't care less what he did. Although this was far from her reality, it dominated his. With testosterone therapy she started to become sexual again, and the marriage, which had been strong, was restored. All could have easily been lost, and for many men there is no way to move past the lack of sexual interest, even if temporary.

HYSTERECTOMIES AND SEXUAL LIBIDO

There is an increasing awareness that many hysterectomies may be unnecessary, and yet this continues to be the second most prevalent surgery in the United States. A survey showed that one-third of American women have had their uterus *and* ovaries removed—often before the age of fifty. In many of these cases, these women were out of balance hormonally and *perhaps* could have avoided surgery if their biochemistry was first balanced. Unfortunately, such is not the way of American medicine today.

Surgical menopause occurs when the ovaries are removed or damaged during surgery. According to Dr. Northrup, approximately one in

every four American women will enter menopause due to surgery, usually meaning by hysterectomy (surgical removal of all or part of the
uterus), which also frequently includes an oophorectomy (surgical removal of the fallopian tubes and ovaries). Any surgery affecting the
pelvic region can potentially damage the ovaries or impair their function.[3]

Many women report diminished sexual response following a hysterectomy. I have witnessed women in despair following what they came
to perceive as an unnecessary hysterectomy. I have heard doctors deny
that this is possible, but I have seen it many times.

Vivienne came to our office at age forty-eight, a year after a hysterectomy, due to having numerous cysts and very painful periods for
years. She had since lost all sexual desire. She said the change had been
instantaneous and enormous. Her doctor told her that it was mostly in
her head and that the surgery had nothing to do with her sexual appara-
tus. But based on our observations, that is untrue, because sexuality is
fundamentally about chemistry. Her hormonal output was enormously
reduced as a result of the surgery, and it was not properly balanced
afterward.

Vivienne was somewhat masculine and dominant by nature. She was
attractive and a little boyish looking; she had a straight-up-and-down
figure commonly seen in women who are low in estrogen. In her younger years she was androgen dominant, meaning that she had lower than
average estrogen levels and higher than average testosterone levels.
This had first been treated medically with drugs, as her doctor believed
that her polycystic ovaries (creating a syndrome known as PCOS) were
due to too much testosterone (without looking at other factors); the
symptoms were acne and excessive hair growth on her face and and
other unwanted areas. Her doctor put her on a drug to lower insulin
levels, as insulin resistance is often a factor in PCOS. These types of
drugs suppress insulin production in the liver and supposedly lead to a
reduction in the clinical aspects of PCOS but do not address the underlying hormonal imbalances.[4] When we tested her a year following her
surgery, she was found to have low levels of both testosterone and
estradiol. These low levels can create a precipitous decline emotionally,
along with other disturbing symptoms.

She was angry, weepy, and lacked the energy necessary to creatively
manage her anger. Estrogen and testosterone were badly needed: estro-

gen for her dark moods and feelings of regret (mostly over having had the surgery), and testosterone for uplifting sadness and increasing her sense of self-esteem and libido.

She found intercourse very painful; her new doctor explained that the low estrogen actually caused a condition called vaginismus, a sustained contraction of vaginal muscles that makes sex very difficult.[5]

Low estradiol also creates dryness; this causes pain when penetration is attempted as the muscles tighten further in anticipatory pain. Her husband took it personally as a rejection. Further, she was exhausted, had headaches, and was dry all over, including her eyes.

She responded beautifully to transdermal estrogen as well as extra estriol (E3) capsules inserted vaginally until she started to self-lubricate. We also had her use a transdermal testosterone cream. A small amount of testosterone can be very powerful; in her case, 1 mg was sufficient. Some women use testosterone only once a day as it can affect sleep; other women find using the cream before 5 p.m. does not affect sleep and allows for greater energy in the evening. Although it took a while to balance her hormones, she has continued to thrive sexually and in terms of her self-awareness and self-esteem.

Another interesting case involved a woman who was quite a powerful force and had an excellent career in psychiatry. Brilliantly educated, Joan had rested on her Ivy League laurels for years. She had a thriving medical practice, then after her marriage, she worked part time as a therapist from her suburban Boston home.

As time passed, her marriage failed and her career, which had been languishing, faltered. Younger, more aggressive women came up and began making their mark. The thing that struck me about Joan was how despondent she was over what she had lost: a career she had not enjoyed for a long time, and a marriage she had known was on weak ground for many years. When the reality hit her—when she realized she no longer wanted to be a therapist and when she saw that her husband was truly a jerk, she had a very difficult time, and her self-esteem plummeted. These life events are often congruent with a loss of hormones, notably in this case, testosterone. Her gynecologist had been a great believer in estrogen and kept her on a lower dose, even after the Women's Health Initiative findings in 2002 had many of his colleagues taking women off completely. Had she gone off the estrogen, her depression would have reappeared, and this, combined with her drop in self-worth, would have been much worse.

We started her on 1 mg of testosterone twice a day, and within weeks her sense of humor returned. Life, while still not easy, actually had room for possibilities. So many women after menopause, whether surgically induced or not, tell us similar stories. The drop in self-esteem is real and piercing. Aging is hard enough on women, and the lack of this most critical hormone makes the process so much more difficult. After six months she started dating again. She also started looking at other work options in psychiatric research and was seeing more possibilities for herself rather than living in resignation.

Another case involving testosterone is very different. Rosalie was a client at our clinic for many years. When we first met her, she had the flattest affect in her voice of any woman I had ever met. She sounded so defeated from years of depression. She had extremely low testosterone, DHEA, and estrogen. Interestingly, it was the addition of testosterone that made the biggest difference in her particular type of depression. The flatness was a major symptom; she never got anxious (she had good progesterone levels), but she felt resigned and hopeless. Women (and men) with this kind of depression live as if they already know the outcome to life. Rose suffered silently a good deal of the time; she thought her family would not think she was so sad if she did not talk about it. In fact, the worst thing about this type of mood disorder is that it is intrinsically linked to "anger turned inward," and she was often feeling angry but too down to deal with it. Testosterone made a difference in her sense of life *and* noticeably in her self-esteem. She felt confident in being a woman and in her ability to somehow break through the inertia she had been feeling for so long.

TESTOSTERONE IN MIDDLE-AGED MEN

As men age their testosterone levels decrease as their estrogen levels increase! This can make very tough guys turn sappy and sentimental as they get older. The rising estrogen makes them less aggressive, and they start to get "breasty"—soft in the chest, as well as in their emotional world. This is generally not such a good thing. Women want men to remain cool, stable, and steadfast, even as they learn to be more accessible and vulnerable as part of becoming more whole human beings, psychologically. The effects of decreasing testosterone levels are similar for men and women, though because testosterone is a male hormone, these effects have much greater intensity and are of primary importance for men.

Men need small amounts of estrogen just as women need small amounts of testosterone. Unfortunately, most men are prone to estrogen excess and testosterone deficiency as they approach middle age. The regulatory mechanism that keeps these systems in check can get stuck as they age. An enzyme called aromatase inhibits testosterone function by converting available testosterone to estrogen. According to Eugene Shippen, an expert in testosterone, estrogen derived from aromatase activity actually displaces testosterone at the receptor sites.[6]

To counter this, aromatase inhibitors can be used (small amounts of progesterone can be used for this purpose, and also there are other inhibitory molecules added at compounding pharmacies). These molecules allow testosterone to do its job without converting into estrogen during the natural "oxidative" or "rusting" process of aging. The bottom line is that there needs to be a delicate balance so that the person, male or female, feels balanced, without too much aggression or too little assertiveness.

There is a wonderful cartoon showing a woman, hands on her hips, shouting at a man slumped in front of the television, saying, "You know, in some cultures, the man does things." Her aggression is obvious—she has too much testosterone! And he has too little, he is just there; no action or will is evident.

Muriel, an aggressive fifty-two-year-old woman, is a great example of androgen (male hormone) dominance. As an adolescent, she was somewhat insecure, not very pretty, and not particularly gifted academically. Instead of being a "shrinking violet," she became more aggressive and bullying, and gentler girls generally avoided her. She was head of a clique of similar girls. Her college years were unremarkable, and she had a few unsuccessful relationships. In her midthirties she married an older wealthy man, who had made his money by somewhat unsavory means. Interestingly, her worst tendencies during adolescence became dominant as she approached midlife and her hormones started to change; she became an aggressive, social-climbing, midlife woman, now with the prestige, in her own mind, of new wealth. But she was not happy. Finally, one day her son, a college student, confronted her about how he saw his parents' obsession with appearance. He was finding their lifestyle increasingly shallow and lacking in meaning and purpose. Muriel had thought her son at least liked and respected her, and this revelation forced her, at menopause, to look in the mirror with different eyes. She entered therapy. Her psychologist was skilled and insightful; she was referred for an evaluation to a doctor who worked with bioidentical hormones and eventually ended up seeing a colleague of mine. I was asked to work with her, also.

The blood tests were a revelation: what showed up was a pattern of male-dominant hormones: she had high levels of testosterone, 98 ng/dl, and DHEA, 160 ug/dl, and very low female hormones: estradiol of 32 pg/nl and progesterone of 0.3 ng/ml. This meant that her male hormones were overwhelming her female hormones. She had never taken female hormones. She had not taken testosterone; however, she had ordered DHEA after reading an article about it in a health magazine. Knowing nothing about her own hormones, she had bought over-the-counter DHEA at a health food store, and she proceeded to take a strong dose (25 mg capsules), which for her was truly excessive. This is much higher than most women need; we have found that 5 to 10 mg is usually sufficient. We also continue to think the less oral use of hormones, the better, as there is less liver involvement. Sometimes oral hormones are all right, but it is not our preferred delivery method.

We use physiologic dosing—not mega dosing. Our goal is to get women back into balance rather than to make older women look or act like teenage girls. The doctors I work with try not to underprescribe or overprescribe.

Muriel had started taking the DHEA for fatigue, although she was already tense and irritable. The DHEA put her further out of balance and made her more irritable. When we saw her, we took her off all DHEA (months later she could take a small amount, about 2.5 mg) and put her on a compounded cream of female hormones, used twice daily. These were the molecules her body was starved for. She became less irritable and defensive. Therapy proved to be hard for her; there was much she really did not want to observe, mainly that her issues with her husband were really about marrying him for his lifestyle, not because she loved him. In fact, they really didn't like each other very much. But she became less aggressive and stopped continually blaming everyone else for her issues.

Muriel had very high testosterone levels relative to estrogen, and her anger was internalized and seething. Yet, as in Rosalie's case, a small dose of female hormones was the turning point in her getting better. While testosterone can be wonderful for women (it is the molecule for self-esteem for midlife women), it needs to be balanced by estrogen. If it becomes a dominant molecule, certain issues develop. These can be obvious physical issues such as POC (polycystic ovaries), or they can be deep internal and emotional issues, such as anger turned inward. This is a major root of depression and can lead to other serious problems.

Ellie was married to a verbally abusive man. For many years, and most of her marriage, she tailored her behavior to suit others. Patricia Evans brilliantly describes the verbal abuser in her groundbreaking work *The Verbally Abusive Relationship*. In this relationship, the abuse was in the marriage, and its source was her husband. For many years he demanded sex three times a day. This was his way of being in charge and making sure the little woman did her job—taking care of him. For a man like this the woman is not real, she is only there as his object. Ellie was invisible and suffered in silence. She became a handmaiden to her husband and a compliant, available woman in all of her relationships, including with her children, who took advantage of her and expected her to do their bidding. Her four children thought she existed for them. What happened to this woman's self-esteem as well as her mental and subsequently physical well-being?

One daughter with four children wanted to return to work and assumed her mother would be the caretaker, as she had always been. Finally, Ellie rebelled and said no, telling her daughter that she wanted more time for herself. She took a huge risk by rocking the boat of the family system this way. Had she done so sooner, maybe she could have thrived more emotionally in all areas.

Shortly after this, she developed serious cervical cancer. According to Louise Hay in her groundbreaking mind/body book *You Can Heal Your Life*, women who get ovarian or cervical cancer may have deep feelings of being unable to claim life for themselves.[7] Of course, other factors must be present, but the emotional soup was ripe. Because of her husband's excessive sexual demands early in their marriage, and at a time when such things were not routinely looked for, Ellie had been repeatedly exposed to human papillomavirus (HPV).

HPV is a virus that occurs as two different types, often referred to as "low risk" (wart causing) or "high risk" (cancer causing), based on whether they put a person at risk for cancer. In 90 percent of cases, the body's immune system clears the HPV infection naturally within two years. This is true of both high-risk and low-risk types. However, if the virus does not clear, then it becomes chronic, and the woman becomes vulnerable to cervical cancer and other related problems.

There are excellent papers documenting the role of di-indole methane, commonly known as DIM, thwarting the development of HPV. DIM contains a molecule called indole-3-carbinol, a potent agent that increases the good estrogens relative to estrone.[8] DIM is commonly found in the cabbage family of vegetables, such as cauliflower, broccoli, and cabbage; women who eat these regularly get this natural protection from their diet.

Ellie went through some traditional treatment and died after a relatively short duration. She was sick for only three months, and she was overwhelmed with starting to look at issues that she had long avoided. Although there was much sadness at her death, one has to wonder what this family was thinking all those years. Her husband was undone—"beside himself" is a good expression here. He had been so utterly dependent on his wife that he could barely function. However, in many ways, he had always been "beside himself," because he shifted emotional responsibility to his wife rather than looking at his own ways of dealing with issues. She carried the burden, and it destroyed her will to live.

I have scientist colleagues who think that mood is strictly biochemical. I do not. I believe it is a many-sided and varied discourse in the dance of being human. There is a whole world to depth psychology— quite synergistic, yet at the same time, independent of biochemistry.

I have a client who has struggled with her sexuality for her entire marriage. Lara's husband did not physically abuse her, but he was unavailable emotionally, which left her feeling very lonely. He simply could not give much, or he would not. How is one to know? Many of the women I see with these issues do not wish to rock the boat of at least being a couple.

This is the context in which I held my work with her. What did she want? She said she wanted to stay in her marriage, but she had pretty much given up on ever finding passion there again. He seemed to have no desire to rekindle his desire or desirability. He enjoyed sex and wished she did more, but she had rarely had a desire for him for years.

It is not my job to advise these women on what to do—but we do open up many conversations for possibilities, and I try to guide women to continue with the right therapist. The mood issues that we address with nutrients and hormones are ultimately a way to allow women to look at the crucial issues of their lives: Does she stay in an emotionally flat marriage or start to look at another way of living?

In Lara's case she had very, very low levels of all hormones when we tested her. She had been on thyroid medication for years and recently had a new medication added to include T3 as well. This had no impact on her weight, although sometimes it can help with weight loss.

Even with these low hormone levels, she had probably long tended toward hormonal imbalance with too much aldosterone and testosterone and DHEA. She was insulin resistant, had PCOS, and felt aggressive much of the time.

Getting more female hormones into the equation helped her tendency toward "resignation depression" a great deal: after about six weeks on estrogen, she stopped assuming that things would not, or could not, ever change. At that time, she was able to use a small amount of additional testosterone to help with her libido.

Unfortunately, it did not increase much. Her issues with her husband were both objective and subjective, the way humans view each other. She was simply not attracted to him. Hormones, on her end, could not make him someone else. Our work has now shifted and is focused on helping her become more whole so that she is able to tolerate her emotional world, whatever is going on.

TESTOSTERONE: THE MOOD MOLECULE OF SELF-ESTEEM

By way of review, as women age and their hormone levels decline, they lose their physical and psychological balance. Testosterone can help restore skin tone, libido, and a sense of assertiveness. According to The Women's Health Connection,[9] proper treatment with testosterone has a wonderful influence for both sexes on:

1. energy and overall well-being
2. strength and stamina
3. ability to perform physically demanding tasks
4. bone density
5. mood, confidence, self-esteem, motivation
6. ability to focus
7. libido and sexual function

I have heard certain physicians recommend testosterone be applied internally to women in order to stimulate sexual appetite. This is not necessary as testosterone absorbed from the skin via compounded gels or creams (our preference) is easily absorbed.

Until recently women—and men—had only the option of synthetic (altered) methyltestosterone, and it has had deleterious side effects in each sex—it is too strong and not the right molecule.

The focus of my work now, along with my physician partner, Dr. Chris Martinez, is finding balance as women age, and we do think women of any age should have balanced hormones for optimal physical and mental health. Bioidentical testosterone helps with lean muscle mass, better metabolic rate, better memory, and increased libido. Testosterone in tiny amounts has helped so many women. We have found quite small amounts wonderfully restorative. If, however, women have too much testosterone relative to their female hormones—and this can happen in women who are not even on hormone supplementation—then androgen (male hormone) dominance develops. These women may become hairier, insulin resistant (more vulnerable to diabetes and other disorders), and more aggressive. Generally, we tell women that if they become aggressive without first becoming assertive, then they are taking too high a dose. The goal is to find a reasonable and rational self-expression without being shrill, defiant, or masculine. We have seen many, many women with low testosterone and a smaller percentage with too high a level relative to their female hormones. *It is the balance among hormones that is critically important.*

THE DHEA-CORTISOL CONNECTION

It is now well established that chronic stress leads to an outpouring of cortisol, and with that, a gradual depletion of DHEA. Over time, this hormonal imbalance can lead to hardening of the arteries, thinning bones, increasing waistline girth, and impaired functioning of the immune system.

High cortisol levels also lead to an increase in blood sugar. In response, more insulin needs to be secreted from the pancreas to clear the sugar from the blood and shepherd it into the cells. In chronic situations, alternating high and low blood sugar levels ensues, and eventually the body becomes less sensitive to insulin.

This phenomenon is commonly known as metabolic syndrome or syndrome X. Several detrimental effects of this syndrome include weight gain and obesity, increases in cholesterol and triglyceride levels, and a rise in blood pressure. Adult onset diabetes also can result. There is a strong relationship to other contributing factors of metabolic syndromes as discussed earlier, such as polycystic ovaries or PCOS. Chronic high levels of cortisol can also impair the immune response. The inability to fight infections leads to a higher susceptibility to colds and flu. [10]

Personally, I saw the wonders of restoring DHEA and lowering cortisol this past winter. Four years of stress following the illness and eventual loss of my husband had weakened my immune system to the point at which I got the flu quite badly. Previously, when I would feel something coming on, I could usually avert it, but not this time. And then I got shingles, a painful debilitating response to a weakened immune system. Shingles occurs when the varicella or chicken pox virus, having lain dormant for decades, comes back to life.

My cortisol levels had gotten very high over the previous months, and my DHEA levels had plummeted. I had continued on my hormones, but my prescription contained too little DHEA to compensate for the rising cortisol. I had been focusing on my depleted primary estrogen levels (estradiol or E2) and ignoring other factors. While my estrogen levels were extremely low, the biggest issue was my lowered immune response because the elevated cortisol overshadowed everything.

I have seen wonderful things start to happen when the person stops the downward spiral of negativity by choice. This is when life can transform, when we assume the role of creator in our own glories and messes. But when the body is exhausted and there is not enough DHEA, the primal instincts of manifesting strength and effective action often vanish. I simply had arrived at the bottom of four years of trauma—the first of which was my beloved husband getting sick, and then his death, and I no longer knew how to make it all work again.

Today I was feeling low all morning. Often mornings have been hard for me since my husband's death, but I had been so much stronger lately. I had taken our son to the airport off to a new phase of his life, and I want him to be free and thrive. But I was missing him terribly and he had just left! Even our dog was low, too.

Then, while working a bit later, I realized that I had not used any testosterone that day, as I had taken my son to the airport so early, and I was feeling the symptoms of low testosterone: flat energy, indecisive, uncertainty about everything. I applied the cream, and I felt it work within the hour.[11] Again, my working premise is that if women have the correct balance of hormones, the moods and emotions that are part of the dance of aging are easier.

After my husband's untimely death at age fifty-seven three years ago, I read everything that appealed to me on grief—many, many books. Books have always been a source of solace for me. It took a while before I could stop doing all I could to heal and to allow time for reflection. One of the best books I read was by Joyce Carol Oates, *A Widow's Story*, a riveting book.[12] It was also all about the author and her experience. I determined that in writing this book, I would use opportunities to bring some of my experience alive in the hope that I could guide the reader to a better understanding of many of these issues.

As I looked back on the year before Jesse got sick, I now see changes I might have been alert to. Was this denial? I always thought I paid exquisite attention to my husband. Was it denial on my part or his? I assume both.

Jesse was an extremely vital man. He was the most wonderful man I had ever known, and he was physically beautiful, rugged, and all too human. He was prone to periods of self-deprecation and pretty deep periods of sadness. We healed old wounds together, and most of his old darkness went away. I believe it resurfaced when he got sick.

About a year or so before, I now remember he fell back into some old ways of speaking that had not been present for years. Often, he was tired, which I attributed to his working too much. We had a beautiful romantic life and a passionate sexual one.

Then he withdrew. He would tell me that "you are the love of my life, now and ever, but sexually I just can't seem to find the way." We both figured in time it would be all right again. We were still young. I avoided going there, and I tried to do everything possible to assure myself and him that we would be fine; there was enormous love and passion always, even when we were not making love a lot the way we always had.

Later, of course, the pieces of the puzzle fit together, and we would both come to realize that his declining interest in sex was an early symptom of other imbalances in his body. I grieved him deeply and profoundly. I also have grieved my own lack of vision and foresight, things I thought I had some mastery of. So, to experience the decline of our sexual life when we loved each other as much as before was very hard. In time, I guess life makes sense. I am waiting.

7

EMOTIONS AND RELATIONSHIPS

The great epochs of our lives are at the points where we gain courage
to rebaptize our badness as the best in us.
—Friedrich Nietzsche

I have a lovely memory of being with my father at a great old Jewish
deli when I was a young girl. An elderly couple came in, sat down and
proceeded to . . . not speak. Finally, the woman, in the age-old attempt
to relate, said, "So, what'll you have?" The old gent said, "I'll have what
I'll have, and you'll have what you'll have."

That was the end of conversation. I think of that scene sometimes as
I witness couples unable to communicate. How does communication
get so frozen? In conscious couples marriage becomes an opportunity
to heal the deep issues we all bring forth from childhood. In unconscious people, one or both people play at the eternal power struggle:
who is dominant? Who has bigger secrets, more control, which ultimately kills intimacy and the desire to connect? The truth is that people
bring their ancestors, children, and much old baggage to midlife relationship issues. And sometimes men and women see each other's baggage rather differently. Then if you throw changing hormones into the
mix, it becomes even more complicated. Women are always aware of
the strong web of emotions and the fragile threads that lie within, and
when women feel destabilized in their moods by the natural hormonal
changes of midlife, this can contribute to even more anxiety for them.

The issues women tell us about repeatedly have to do with relationship matters and self-esteem issues, the latter being the basis of a strong

container for the ego. Only when that is intact can one give up trying to prove they are okay.

One of the biggest differences between men and women is that female brains respond to emotional patterns differently: women are generally more process oriented, while men tend to be more goal oriented. For women, conversation is extremely critical when they are in trouble: by talking in a safe space the brain actually starts to rewire itself. The right conversations, along with biochemical balancing, can inhibit neurons, which in turn calms the emotions.

Men usually want to make their partner feel better or avoid conflict, often with less conversation, which creates further conflict as the woman needs to be in the space of conversation and conflict to move through and get past it. John Bradshaw once said, "The way out is through."[1] This is vitally important for women, as their daily well-being is consistently impacted by mood and their moods are directly affected by their relational world. Men are also deeply moved by love, of course, but it is generally observed that most men can put emotional issues aside by having a beer or distracting themselves in some other more significant way.

Several months ago, I received the following email that was probably a joke, but at the same time it represented an age-old difference between the way that men and women see relationships:

Wife's Diary: Tonight, I thought my husband was acting weird. We had made plans to meet at a nice restaurant for dinner. I was shopping with my friends all day long, so I thought he was upset at the fact that I was a bit late, but he made no comment on it. Conversation wasn't flowing, so I suggested that we go somewhere quiet so we could talk. He agreed, but he didn't say much. I asked him what was wrong. He said, "Nothing." I asked him if it was my fault that he was upset. He said he wasn't upset, that it had nothing to do with me, and not to worry about it. On the way home, I told him that I loved him. He smiled slightly, and kept driving. I can't explain his behavior. I don't know why he didn't say, "I love you, too." When we got home, I felt as if I had lost him completely, as if he wanted nothing to do with me anymore. He just sat there quietly and watched TV. He continued to seem distant and absent. Finally, with silence all around us, I decided to go to bed. About fifteen minutes later, he came to bed. But I still felt that he was distracted, and his thoughts were somewhere else. He fell asleep—I cried. I don't know what to do. I'm almost sure that his thoughts are with someone else. My life is a disaster.

Husband's Diary:

Boat wouldn't start. Can't figure it out.

If men and women live so differently in their relational worlds, how do two people who truly love each other communicate? Certainly excellent books have been written about communication by professors of linguistics such as Deborah Tannen[2] and pop psychologists such as John Gray in *Men Are from Mars, Women Are from Venus*.[3] Knowing we communicate differently helps us to allow for more effective possibilities but does not help the primary issues of how to live within a self that is whole and contained without being ego excessive. What makes one woman plunge into a probable catastrophic relationship and another bide her time no matter how lonely? As we age, hopefully we learn that the ego must have a strong container first, before it can give up pieces that no longer serve it. This is what depth psychologists call making the darkness conscious. I have found repeatedly that the women who have had help balancing their hormones and mood chemistry and have also spent time delving into their own psychological nature move through life passages well, even if problems are currently present. These are deeply connected aspects of the dance of being female and lead to the deepest of feminine attributes often lost in today's culture: the essence is being relational, and the core in intimate relationships is being receptive. Today's women have a great deal of confusion on these issues, and there is suffering because of this.

I have found in our clinical work that when women are overwhelmed by life's emotional passages, their health is affected. Sometimes this shows up in small, irritating ways, such as recurrent headaches or fatigue, though oftentimes it can show up in significant ways that seem irredeemable. As mentioned in the previous chapter, women desperately need the balance of libido strength to create the possibility of options when there seem to be few or none. Often, we have seen that the addition of a small amount of testosterone allows this emotional strength to develop. Women who learn to stay strong in the face of uncommon adversity rise to the occasion, and as they keep learning to reach for that better thinking that can bring a new vision at best, or even an initial sense of relief at least, then new doors open.

Our emotional/relational world impacts our health and well-being, if not always directly, then in nuanced and subtle ways that become more vivid as we learn more about what each of us brings to the table. Relationships reveal us; they do not make us who we are. Many, many women have sat in my office complaining about their relationships and how this impacts their sense of well-being.

A big part of late midlife relational health evolves from first becoming truly whole ourselves; then if we are presented with options we can choose what is best for our journey, knowing that we cannot control all aspects of destiny. Biochemistry is one part of this story; however, there are also many psychological aspects that influence the female psyche. Balanced biochemistry allows women to endure the perils of aging that is new turf for women.

WORDS AS WEAPONS

Women are relational by nature. Patricia Evans writes in her brilliant book *The Verbally Abusive Relationship* about how many people can be verbal abusers. She explains how this is not always self-evident—it may not be an overt or direct statement. Instead, verbal abuse can be subtle, and it is insidious and destructive. If a woman is in a relationship with a verbally abusive man, it can damage her psyche and her health; the two are intertwined in many ways. [4]

Verbal abusers know what they are doing: this is a tool to manipulate and control. The objective of the abuser is to make the woman into his ideal; therefore, any hint of her own essence of individuality that threatens his perception cannot be tolerated. If the woman wants to go to dinner with girlfriends but he had another plan in mind, he will use this against her with statements such as "See, you never put me first," or "I knew you did not care about what I want," which leaves her staggering with the unspoken "but what about what I want?" It does not matter. The unspoken resentment goes into her biology, and she becomes less vital, and often eventually ill. Again, with balanced hormones, notably progesterone, allowing her to contemplate before responding, she can learn about putting her emotional needs ahead of the survival of a relationship.

How women deal with relationship issues affects all aspects of mood. Sadly, what often forces one to face the unworked parts of oneself is the overwhelming loss of a relationship, whether it is a precious relationship, lost through the death of the beloved, or a difficult, toxic relationship that has ended by separation. Unworked depression is often a river that runs through the drama, affecting future outcomes. Dealing with depression involves much more than simply going to therapy; the person must descend deeply into her own psyche and see what remains after facing oneself.

If, at a major midlife crisis when all is apparently lost, perhaps following death or divorce, one can start to see daylight again, there is a new listening, a new perspective.

Relationships, and how we process them, are integral to how healthy we are emotionally, independent of whether one is currently in an intimate primary relationship. Dr. Carl Jung would acknowledge someone who was deep in a time of grief and loss, saying this period in the descent would produce great richness ahead if consciously dealt with.

Gary met Paula at a time when both were newly alone. Gary was coming out of a marriage he had thought was "just fine" until his wife decided she was tired of marriage and of him. He was a big hunk of a guy, larger than life, but his ego was shot down. He had never done any soul searching and could only perceive others in terms of himself.

When he met Paula, who was very attractive and accomplished, they initially sensed possibility. But almost immediately after a couple of good times, he gave off unconscious warnings that his needs and ego would take precedence. Paula quickly became unattracted. Though he was surprised, he did not try to discover why this highly desirable woman had turned away.

Paula had been our client for a long time, and her sense of personal balance was largely linked to the fact that her hormones had been well balanced in her late forties through midfifties; for years she had used natural progesterone during two weeks of formerly harsh PMS, and then she had slowly added a small amount of testosterone for energy and decisiveness. Finally, she had somewhat reluctantly added estrogen, about a year before fully in menopause, as she was having several key symptoms. Most notably she developed very dry skin, started to wrinkle more, and felt a loss of a sense of excitement in her life, as well as brain fog. She had blood levels of less than 30 pg/ml of estrogen, which we considered extremely low. She was a little cautious with estrogen as she knew several women who had breast cancer. However, none of these women had ever used bioidentical hormones. Some had been on standard horse urine estrogen, most with progestins (not real progesterone) and one without any progestin. Others had never used hormones at all.

Paula read extensively, talked with several medical people, and decided to try a small dose of estrogen, not quite as much as we would normally give someone with the symptoms and blood levels she exhibited. Even with this low dose, she felt much better. She quickly realized the small amount of estrogen helped her find and maintain her sense of herself as a woman; therefore, she did not need a man to validate her.

Gary, on the other hand, was another story. He was wounded, and therefore he needed to wound someone else. Many men go from relationship to relationship quickly because they have never learned to grieve. Relationships require some processing when they end, however they end. About ten weeks later he met Kandra, cute and conservative, a lot more predictable, but with no depth. In contrast to Paula, she was not well educated, and she willing to put up with almost anything to be on the arm of this handsome, newly single guy. While she had made some money selling real estate and considered herself an independent woman, she was incredibly needy and codependent. She played all her games, from pouting and adolescent games of attraction, and his undeveloped anima (the feminine unconscious in the male) was so latent, and so very in need of attention, that they quickly became a couple. He was not in love with her, though she professed to be totally in love very quickly (her first big mistake), and he was masterful at withdrawing and making her wonder. Yet they fulfilled each other's saddest, desperate needs. He got to be a "big shot" again, in her eyes; she got to have a guy.

Kandra had a vacuous, smooth face that reflected her lack of depth; she was not arresting, but she had almost nary a single line at age fifty-eight! The repeated injections of anti-aging treatment had frozen her into a cold stare. What she did not disclose to Gary was that she had frequent panic attacks and lived in a state of perpetual anxiety. Her doctor had her taking an antidepressant, and although Kandra would likely have benefited from the calming influence of progesterone, she had no interest in investigating the possibility of bioidentical hormones. She chose to believe instead of explore. In fact, her whole life was about belief, including her ardent attachment to her religious beliefs, and now her newfound god in yet another undeveloped male, Gary. The undeveloped psyche of this new couple was doomed, but each was in it for his or her own reasons, not for love. Neither was capable of genuine intimacy.

Another man, Warren, idolized his wife, Bea, for many years. But she did not love him, and they had not been intimate for years. Bea had been low in estrogen for most of her life, which resulted in her being tall and thin, the very elongated bone structure developed because of genetics and low primary estrogen. When there is not enough estrogen in the teen years, menses occurs later than average, and the bones become long and thin due to the fact that there is not enough estrogen to promote closure of the bone. Had Bea been given estrogen early enough, perhaps a few years before menopause, she might have been able to strengthen her bones, and her persona; as she was in her later sixties both were brittle.[5] She was a withheld type of woman, who was intriguing to a certain kind of man—one who thinks he can get blood from a stone. Of course, this can be said in the inverse as well: some men seem intriguing to certain women, unless or until the discovery is made that there is no one much living there.

BRINGING COUPLES TO CONSCIOUSNESS

Relationships that are conscious have *He, She,* and *We.* There are three short books by these titles by the wonderful writer, Robert Johnson. These books talk about the need for each third to have its own strong identity.[6] According to Johnson, relationships have a life of their own. This is crucial in stepfamilies, or newly formed families. Sometimes, children or relatives from someone's past presume that they "own" the person who has fallen newly in love, and often a great love will bring out the demons. Instead of trying to understand what this rage says about its owner, it is projected upon the new love. The healthy couple will not allow this; each must maintain his/her own boundaries, which can be quite distinct.

Jamie found the love of his life, finally—they were both in their forties, each with one child. His daughter, who was very attached to him, did not want this and was hell-bent on destroying this truly great love. As she had no power to do so, her rage intensified and was projected upon the woman. It would have been projected on any self-contained healthy woman; her rage was actually not personal. Jamie became healthier as he psychically separated from his daughter, a very crucial step for him. However, the woman, June, had to protect herself and their relationship.

Jamie felt the conflict and felt sad about it, but he had found joy. The woman he loved was very balanced, calm, and kind, but she would not be dumped on; she was no doormat, and had done years of work on her own issues. She knew she had found what was right for her. While Jamie's daughter tried to make her look bad whenever possible, June found her that keeping her hormones balanced helped enormously. When she could not sleep she used more progesterone, magnesium, and sometimes anxiety-control nutrients, as she started obsessing negatively: what if Jamie left her because of this? In truth, he had never thought of this. June found extra progesterone astounding in its quieting-the-mind effect.

Over time he saw how his daughter was so much like his mother, unwilling to process anything, but great at projection and blame. June initially thought it was her obligation to encourage this endless, hopeless "trying" to integrate this difficult daughter, who was so cold and harsh toward her and them. The big lesson learned for her: Not all relationships are transformable, nor should they be.

My client in this case was the woman, and I often wondered about Jamie's daughter. She was most likely low in estrogen (she had the telltale body type of tall, elongated bones). When mood disorders exist strongly in women with low estrogen, the tendency is toward depression, and if unchecked, rage. Anger turned inward manifests as dark depression, and if turned outward it is rage projected on whomever is the target. It is unconscious anger, as it really does not understand itself. Could some of the behavioral issues have been addressed in adolescence in a manner that produced a more effective early entry into womanhood? Then perhaps life could have been so much easier for her father, the woman he loved, and the girl herself. However, she was not interested in any inquiries that suggested she was less than perfect; alas, this was her journey, not theirs.

WOMEN ARE GETTING HEALTHIER—WHAT ABOUT MEN?

Michael Meade talks about the unconscious anger of so many men and the unhealed wounds they carry around and bring full bore into their adult relationships. Many of these men are infantile emotionally, and the women they live with are similarly arrested. Robert Moore, the Jungian scholar and professor, wrote *King, Warrior, Magician, Lover*,[7] a wonderful jewel of a book on the four components of the male psyche that must be present for a man to become whole. Most men never venture into the archetypal to learn about the psyche and also to learn that perhaps not everything psychologically directed is about them. Most do not do the work to become self-sustaining and self-contained. They look to others for validation. This is one reason why so many women are unhappy in their relationships; they are trying to be in relationships with men they feel a need to protect psychologically. Sometimes I have the sense that there is an unspoken complicity in many couples: the man takes care of the physical world, and the woman takes care of emotion. Ultimately this leaves a kind of stagnation, as no growth happens in the couple. I have observed this many times in couples I have worked with, often in conjunction with one of the therapists I refer to.

In the work world, women try to find their way and are indeed often mentored. But I often see a toll on relationships unless there is true mutual support. In many professions, in order to excel, women think that they need to become more masculine in their way of being. As an example, a man I know told a woman who was attracted to him when they met for the first time: "I like direct conversation." Later she realized that she wished she had said her truth: that sometimes she did not like direct conversation but preferred deep, circuitous, nonlinear discussions that are more about living and exploring in the Tao, being in the present. She felt she gave up something important by allowing him to set the tone of the relationship, and she decided that she would not make that mistake again so readily. Often, women feel a sense of loss when they abdicate their instinctive lives too quickly. Of course, I as a woman scientist have a reverence for logic and science, but not always in my personal life. Good science can be counterintuitive. Trusting my instincts in my inner life is something I hold as precious.

The energy of the Puer (Peter Pan)—the boy who refuses to grow up, is fairly pervasive in the United States today. Maturity is not a function of how much stuff one has or how many children one sires. Often this strutting kind of boy/man became arrested in his psychological development long ago, following his parents' divorce or some other trauma when he unconsciously decided he had to "be a man." But the problem is that he decided he had to be a man outwardly without ever becoming a man inwardly. This has to be earned in the process of life itself.

IMPORTANCE OF APPROPRIATE FATHER ENERGY

In my clinical work, I see over and over again how unhealthy father energy affects women. Linda Leonard writes beautifully about this in *The Wounded Woman*. She suggests that there are two different types of wounds the father can inflict on his daughters: the too-distant father or the too-involved father. The latter type often shows up in men who take on too much in order to prove themselves, then when divorce happens they compensate by being overly close to their daughters. This type of man idealizes his daughters the way his wife would not allow— she wanted a grown-up love—and these girls become damaged by too much closeness and projection.[8] According to Linda Schierse Leonard and other prominent analysts, these girls assume too much power with men inaccurately, and it affects future relating skills. A man needs to assess proper emotional as well as the obvious physical boundaries with his daughters; the ideal is a healthy, loving, contained relationship, where the daughter's role is never confused with a lover or spouse. In fact, this is the determination of a healthy father-daughter relationship.

NONROMANTIC RELATIONSHIPS FOR WOMEN

Relationships for women take on many forms and can be very complex. In addition to romantic male/female relationships, the intensity of woman/woman relationship can be tenuous. I am referring primarily to non-lesbian female friendships here. So many women compete for male attention that sometimes the illusion of sisterhood is just that. Women use the same tools to manipulate other women as they do with men. Once it was simpler to say, "Beware of a woman you see betraying another woman with a man; she will do this in female friendships as well." Yet the richness and depth of female friendship can also be priceless to women. I have seen examples that have shown me how much uncertainty plays into our roles in relationships today. For example, if a woman is attracted to a man who is clearly unhappy with his current relationship, should she explore this or leave it alone? It is not always so black-and-white.

COUPLES GROWING TOGETHER—OR APART

In my work, often it is the woman who initially comes to me for help with her relationship. I try not to make assumptions about how couples function and what the core of the relationship is, as there are so many pieces that I cannot see as an outside observer. Sometimes when I am seeing a woman I will ask her how she thinks her husband would assess her emotional world if I asked him. Sometimes I ask if these men can come in for a joint session. With full permission from both partners, this is often a deep conversation in which more can come forth for me to work with biochemically. When emotional issues get opened in my space, the goal is then to refer these women and their partner to the right therapist; we often all continue working together. I make changes in hormones and supplements as different patterns emerge.

Recently, a woman whom I had been working with for two years came in to talk about some changes. She had met a man, and she was so glad she had her libido and sexual energy available. But he had some health problems, and they had just had their first frank conversation; he was afraid that her strong vitality might be more than he could measure up to after some things he was dealing with. She told me this was a space that must be treaded carefully, as she did not want to fall into reassuring him at the expense of her own needs and happiness. On the other hand, she really wanted to explore this relationship.

I continue to see amazing shifts in women when they have intact self-esteem and connection to their core selves inside or outside of their primary relationship. Looking through my biochemical lens, I see that this happens best when women are hormonally in balance. The healing energy of conscious love is what helps people become whole and alive and magnificent. The darkest times can be gotten through in this way, and life does indeed surprise us poignantly, and without warning!

8

DISEASES OF AGING/ADVENTURES IN AGING

Modern medicine has extended the average life span significantly, but one has to wonder, at what cost? There are so many diseases out there now that were unheard of one hundred years ago. These are the so-called diseases of aging. While our Western medical establishment prides itself on extending the average life span of individuals, many times it is at the expense of quality of life. In this chapter, I discuss many of these diseases, and I offer some insight and alternatives to the traditional approaches that most doctors today subscribe to. I also talk about how hormones fit into the anti-aging discourse.

> "IF"
> By Rudyard Kipling
> If you can keep your head when all about you
> Are losing theirs, and blaming it on you,
> If you can trust yourself when all men doubt you,
> But make allowance for their doubting too;
> If you can wait and not be tired by waiting. . . .

The beginning of this epic poem by Rudyard Kipling speaks volumes to the courage a scientifically or medically credible person must have in order to go "outside the box" and see things with a different perspective. Thus we arrive at "Diseases of Aging," which may more aptly be called "Adventures in Aging: How to Get Older without Falling Victim to the Dark Side of the Medical Establishment and Take Many Unnecessary Drugs."

Suppose that a third of the drug arsenal in the United States is comprised of truly life-saving or just generally good, helpful drugs (aspirin would fall in here, as well as some of the best biological medicines, based on treating the genetics of cancer). Another third of the drug arsenal are in the gray zone. Maybe they help sometimes, maybe they often don't but they do not do much harm, or maybe they don't often cause iatrogenic (doctor- or drug-induced) medical mishaps. The last third are harmful, and they have been pushed through the FDA too fast for safety concerns to be validated. Where does that leave the average person? I refer the reader to the difficult but excellent book by Siddhartha Mukerjee, *The Emperor of All Maladies*, in which he traces the origins of major cancer therapies. It is easy to see where the phrase *practicing medicine* comes from after reading this.[1]

Drug promotion is so misleading in medicine, most notably in oncology. Loved ones are told that some promising new drug costing many thousands of dollars—often out of pocket—could slow the progression of the cancer. And for some cancers, traditional therapies do work some of the time. Yet when the statistics are studied, often the prolongation of life is minimal and the quality of life is dismal due to the disease combined with truly awful side effects of commonly used drugs.[2]

"OUTSIDE THE BOX": SCIENTIFIC CANCER PROTOCOLS THAT SAVE LIVES

There are many wonderful physicians out there, but in general I think the cancer industry is in dire need of a complete transformation. Cancer is big business, with all those drugs and machines and hundreds of millions of dollars being generated in revenues for various entities.

When a person is diagnosed with cancer, the first response is fear, and the medical environment immediately responds to that with more fear: suggested regimens can be scary, and unanswered questions abound. Most cancer patients lose some of their vitality, and many never fully regain it after an onslaught of treatments that may involve surgery, chemotherapy, and radiation. Once life is damaged at the cellular level from an assault on DNA from radiation and chemotherapy cocktails, full vitality may feel as though it's been lost forever. Of course, if there is any hope for life, people do what they must to possibly survive. The questions arise when the options that might be most helpful at a critical juncture are not widely accessible or known. Why is that?

Some physicians that think outside the box have been ostracized from the medical establishment, primarily because they threaten the "business" of the cancer industry. Dr. Stanislaw Burzynski is one of them. He is an internationally recognized physician and scientist who has devoted his whole life to cancer research. Burzynski Clinic has been treating thousands of cancer patients from all over the world for over forty years. Dr. Burzynski is a pioneer in cancer research, and he is known worldwide for discovering antineoplastons, which act as molecular switches to turn off cancer cells without destroying normal cells. Specifically, what Burzynski and his colleagues look at is twofold:

1. How to make one's own body responsive to turning off oncogenes (cancer-promoting genes) and using drugs and nutrients to help someone make their own missing antineoplastons. These important peptide molecules have gone missing when someone develops cancer. These are the molecules that turn off cancer-promoting genetics.
2. Using drugs to target the DNA; for instance, this means that one can have breast cancer and yet actually have the genetic mutation for colon cancer, but in a given individual the marker for colon cancer may show up in the breast. Therefore, the targeted cancer is actually colon cancer.

The treatments involve drugs and strong nutrients, but they are often used "off label" in ways that are consistent with good science and medicine but are considered experimental. These novel approaches are often not covered by insurance because the way the drugs are used is still considered experimental, even though they have been rigorously followed in clinical trials and even though they save lives.

Dr. Burzynski's protocols are considered a threat to the entire cancer industry. If his protocols were followed, it would mean a massive reorganization of a multi-billion-dollar industry. According to Dr. Julian Whitaker, Burzynski's antineoplaston therapy is a successful alternative to traditional chemotherapy drugs, which threatens the pharmaceutical industry in huge ways. Dr. Whitaker says:

Without exception, all the oncologists I talked to about Dr. Burzynski were scornful and hostile. Twenty-five years of practicing unconventional medicine did not prepare me for what I discovered. Delving into attitudes, actions, and beliefs of modern oncologists was like opening a box of cereal and finding it full of worms. They just don't care. The question I kept asking was why, and the answer to that question gradually began to creep out: Dr. Burzynski's discovery threatens one of the largest and most lucrative industries in the history of mankind, the cancer treatment industry.

All those radiation machines and doctors who run them

All those chemotherapy drugs and the doctors who prescribe them

All those so called studies that just juggle the doses of chemo & radiation, and

All those surgeons who have been flailing at cancer for over 100 years.

Also it is not just about money, it is about strongly held beliefs, beliefs that have meshed with the personality of virtually everyone in the cancer treatment industry, especially the physicians. In short, these beliefs are that cancer can only be treated with therapies that mutilate, poison, or burn the patient, in the hope that they "kill" the cancer. Therefore, each patient who is miraculously cured by Burzynski's nontoxic therapy is not viewed as a breakthrough, or even as something good, but rather as a dangerous messenger of heresy, a terrible threat to their beliefs. Fly to Texas.[3]

The way Burzynski has been treated is appalling—and I see the fear driving this ostracization. He does not fit in, and he threatens the status quo. He was considered an outsider from the oncology establishment and labeled a quack and worse from those threatened by new knowledge. The Texas Medical Board tried to make it impossible for him to practice medicine and to conduct FDA-sanctioned clinical trials for brain cancer. Only recently has he been able to get these stage 111 clinical trials in process.

Not everyone who goes to Burzynski recovers; some die, of course, but statistically many more with "terminal" diagnoses go on to live healthy lives in full remission, or perhaps cured. And many people he has treated—with lousy and acute diagnoses—are back in life fully the following year.

When someone comes along such as Stanislaw Burzynski or a number of others, they are perceived as a threat to the status quo and are derided as "quacks." Someday we may see our current way of treating cancer as archaic, even dangerous. Perhaps we won't, but opening the door to alternative ways of treating cancer may just help save more lives. There are many other excellent doctors working with alternative cancer protocols. A notable doctor is Ron Hunninghake at the Bright Spot for Health Clinic, now called the Riordan Center after the iconoclastic Hugh Riordan, its late founder. They are using megadose vitamin C therapy to treat certain cancers. Under the guidance of the late Hugh Riordan, the center developed an orthomolecular, nutrient-based approach to looking at cancer and all degenerative disease. Hugh Riordan was a great mentor and friend of mine, and I owe him a debt of gratitude. The first time I lectured at the International Society for Orthomolecular Medicine Conference in Toronto, I was too naive to be nervous: I just did what I do best—brought the science alive into the moods of women discourse. He wrote me a letter I treasure in which he said, "I thought your lecture was nothing short of outstanding!" That meant a great deal to me as a young scientist. He and Abram Hoffer are two of the great doctors on whose shoulders I proudly stand.

Christiane Northrup, MD, an eminent physician who has worked extensively on women's life transitions, notably menopause, was a former professor at the University of Vermont School of Medicine, and she speaks about the fear-based medicine surrounding women and cancer in her books and newsletters. To quote from her newsletter of November 2007:

> Here's how I see the traditional medical approach to promoting breast health: See your doctor for a breast exam and have your annual mammogram. If it's normal you can breathe a sigh of relief. . . . Don't worry. You don't have it—yet. But keep coming back because the harder we look, the more we're going to find.

She goes on to say:

> I'm sorry to sound cynical, but I can't help it. Want the truth? Billions of dollars have been spent on breast cancer research (and sadly, different organizations often compete with each other for the same research funds), yet the rate of breast cancer hasn't gone down appreciably.[4]

The focus seems to be more on activity than on accomplishment! The fact is women are more than the sum of their parts; they are more than two breasts constantly on the verge of damaging their life force and well-being.

The foremost premise of our work is that "women are not allergic to their own biology" and that the fear around cancer has led to misinterpretations that are critical in defining how to help women stay healthy, starting with continued use of bioidentical hormones as we age. I continue to see that most cases of gender-based, hormone-linked cancers happen at times in life when women are low in hormones, not at times when hormones are high. Very rarely do pregnant women develop sex-hormone-linked cancer, and they are in a sea of hormones. Theoretically it appears that progesterone acts as a regulator of cellular division: the developing fetus is in a state of controlled cellular division, as contrasted to a tumor gone wild, where there is chaotic proliferation.

I see so many women who are in decline that seems most clearly linked to not having their hormones anymore. I have repeatedly seen the brain fog that becomes a dominant symptom as women age, because they do not have enough of the important estrogen (estradiol, or E2) and their increased fat cells manufacture the less desirable estrogen (estrone, or E1). As estrone rises and estradiol falls, brain fog takes over. The antidote is to increase estradiol to take precedence over estrone. There is no reason why a proper dose of bioidentical hormones would not be appropriate for aging women: this is the ignored demographic. These are the women we must help.

Again we stress that we are not looking for anti-aging or the fountain of youth: this book is about how to age better than most women ever had the chance to do. Very few women have the knowledge to navigate well through this challenging time. We aim to reach women fifty and older, the forgotten ones.

As mentioned earlier in this book, according to Jeffrey Dach, MD, a specialist in bioidentical hormone use, a great deal of confusion exists due to flawed data from a flawed study—The Women's Health Initiative, which was halted in 2002.[5] It is clear that the real culprit is synthetic progestin, not real progesterone and not proper use of estrogen. Synthetic progestin has been shown repeatedly to make women more vulnerable to breast cancer,[6] while progesterone is protective against breast cancer and provides innumerable benefits for female mood issues. Dr. Dach, an innovative crusader for women's proper hormones, calls synthetic progestins monster hormones. This is due to the monstrous side-chains added to the base molecule to make it a saleable, patentable drug. This has hurt many women, and they have aged less well.

In the second arm of the Women's Health Initiative, the women were put on Premarin® (nonbioidentical estrogen only) but not Provera® (synthetic progestin) because all these women in the second half of the study had undergone hysterectomies. Conventional medical thinking has long been to only give progestin to women who had their uterus intact because its purpose is to prevent endometrial cancer; no uterus means no endometrial lining, therefore the general medical thinking is no need for a progestin. However, this is only part of the picture. Real progesterone serves two other major purposes: it is protective against other cancers, and it is the primary calming hormone for women's brains and nervous systems, at all ages. So many women struggle with anxiety linked to hormone depletion, especially progesterone.

Why is it that women have the most cancer when their primary hormones are at their lowest—after menopause—and the least cancer when they are pregnant or at very fertile or optimal biological times of life? Of course, age plays a role as DNA mutations and oxidative stress increase as we age. However, the only women with elevated cancer risk on hormones in the WHI and similar studies were those on synthetic progestins (usually Provera); the women on just Premarin—even though it is not the best estrogen for women—did not have an increase in cancer rates.[7]

Genetics also plays a huge role in cancer, and we are not advocating estrogen for high-risk women, but for the general population there is no more important place to begin rational aging than with bioidentical hormones.

There is an interview in *The Townsend Letter* with Dr. Jonathan Wright by Suzanne Somers; it is titled "Hormones . . . the Backbone of Health and Quality of Life." The premise is that the cancer-protective genes in our bodies lose their potency as our hormone production declines.[8] Ms. Somers states that we should strive for perfect hormonal balance in order to keep cancer at bay. Scientific studies document the protective effect of progesterone and estriol (E3) against breast cancer.[9] Ms. Somers states that Dr. Wright and Dr. Julie Taguchi both feel that bioidentical hormone replacement therapy (BHRT) is protective against cancer and related to favorable gene expression.[10] While I agree with this to a point, I do not believe there is "a perfect balance," but rather, by rationally balancing our hormones we create greater resistance to cancer and other elements of aging and decline. There is, however, no perfect way to avoid cancer.

HEART HEALTH AND MIND/BODY CONNECTIONS

In looking at mind/body connections, we are not blaming the patient for becoming ill—things happen in life, sometimes with seeming randomness. However, our desire is to shed some light on possible emotional patterns constitutive of certain types of illness. Most importantly, the purpose of this book is to help steer women toward other healing approaches, including the emotional descent that accompanies disease.

Jane had a diagnosis of significant heart disease at age forty-eight. She had a supportive network and the willingness to look deeply at issues that had not served her in the past. Unconscious rage in this sweet, petite woman stemmed from the first sense of a bully from a brother who loathed her brightness, and her rage was often misdirected at men she dated. Through therapy, Jane discovered that her sweet, compliant nature actually masked a great deal of anger and aggression. She was very "other-directed," and relationships meant too much to her; when a woman puts her "survival" into a relationship, then she cannot be herself because the self has been swallowed by the duality of the relationship. The submissive, submerged woman has anger that will eventually emerge, one way or another.

She developed heart disease at a relatively young age. Most women do not develop cardiac problems until after menopause; at that point they start catching up to men. Part of this has to do with buildup of iron causing an impact on arterial plaque—after menopause women are not losing iron every month.

More significantly, the loss of estrogen in the form of estradiol creates vascular constriction. Vascular problems are the leading cause of heart disease in women, where cardiac occlusion or congested arteries is the biggest issue for men. Estrogen is the key to keeping arteries healthy in menopausal women. Estrogen has a profound effect on mood as you have been learning in this book; depression, sadness, and heart disease often go hand in hand.

In the December 2012 issue of *Health and Healing* there is important information on how to heal heart disease without the usual trauma of sometimes unnecessary heart surgery. Dr. Whitaker writes about the death of Neil Armstrong, the outstanding American and pioneering astronaut, who died two weeks after bypass surgery. Dr. Whitaker's article went so far as to state that this and many similar surgeries may be unnecessary at best, dangerous at worst. Numerous studies dating back three decades suggest that for some patients, surgical intervention is no more effective than more conservative treatments.[11] These include methods to raise good lipids through dietary sources such as fish oils or vegetable oils such as flax.

Increasing antioxidant protection through various well-established vitamin and nutrient protocols and reducing cardiac inflammatory markers such as C-CRP and homocysteine can be very important to reversing the chemistry associated with heart disease in women. This can be done with B vitamins, such as B12 and folic acid and vitamin B6, and stress reduction and/or meditation-based programs such as those pioneered at the University of Massachusetts by Jon Kabat-Zinn and others.[12]

OSTEOPOROSIS

Osteoporosis is a relatively new disease that has become epidemic because of our increased longevity. As with many other diseases of aging, misinformation abounds, and modern Western medicine has treated the symptoms while failing to understand the underlying causes.

Osteoporosis in women is defined by the World Health Organization (WHO) as "a bone mineral density 2.5 standard deviations below peak bone mass (20-year-old healthy female average) as measured by DXA (Dual energy X-ray absorptiometry)." A bone mineral density between 1.0 and 2.5 standard deviations below peak is considered osteopenia. The term *established osteoporosis* includes the presence of a fragility fracture.

In the human body, bone is continually being remodeled, meaning that bone is being broken down (or "resorbed") and new bone is constantly being synthesized. This process starts before birth and continues throughout a person's lifetime. The underlying mechanism in all cases of osteoporosis is an imbalance between bone resorption and bone formation. In normal bone, this is a constant process, and at any point, up to 10 percent of all bone mass may be undergoing remodeling. In younger years, particularly during adolescence, new bone is synthesized at a faster rate than it is broken down, and as a person approaches adulthood, this becomes more of a steady state. During adulthood, the rate of new bone synthesis gradually slows down, and then in women during menopause, this rate drops precipitously.

Osteoporosis can develop in three ways: 1) inadequate peak bone mass (the skeleton does not develop enough mass and strength during growth); 2) excessive bone resorption (breakdown); or 3) inadequate synthesis of new bone during remodeling. When one of these mechanisms is out of balance, bone is not properly formed and becomes brittle and more susceptible to fracture. While there are many factors that affect this balance, the bone-remodeling process is driven by hormones. Estrogen slows down bone resorption, and progesterone encourages new bone growth. Thus, a drop in the levels of these hormones (such as occurs in menopause) results in bone being broken down at a faster rate, while new bone is being produced a slower rate!

This is a natural process of aging. Every woman goes through this process. Therefore, any fifty- to fifty-five-year-old woman who is in or around menopause will have a bone density significantly less than that of any twenty-year-old healthy female. What this means for women is that based on the WHO definition of osteoporosis "a bone mineral density 2.5 standard deviations below peak bone mass of a 20-year-old healthy female average," *the majority of women will be given a diagnosis of osteoporosis or osteopenia when they are postmenopausal.* However, our working premise is that with bioidentical hormone replacement therapy, this process can be slowed down, and even reversed.

Bone is living tissue, and it is greatly affected by diet and mineral absorption. The primary bone minerals are calcium phosphate, calcium carbonate, and magnesium, while some trace minerals such as boron and selenium are needed in very tiny quantities. Collagen, the primary bone protein, is held in place by a matrix of these minerals.

Hormones, especially the sex hormones, play a supporting role in building better bones throughout a woman's life. Estrogen slows down bone resorption; after menopause bone resorption rates increase, which contributes to more bone loss.[13] It is so important that doctors recommend estrogen for women vulnerable to fractures, but they often neglect real progesterone, especially when there is no uterus involved (women who have had hysterectomies). Progesterone actually starts new bone growth and contributes to bone density and strength. It is now thought that women with accelerated bone loss are also deficient in testosterone as well as estrogen and progesterone. Again, it is a question of balance.[14]

Interestingly, the International Society for Clinical Densitometry has taken the position that a diagnosis of osteoporosis in men under fifty years of age should not be made on the basis of densitometric criteria alone. It also states that for premenopausal women, Z-scores (comparison with age group rather than peak bone mass) should be used, and that the diagnosis of osteoporosis in such women also should not be made on the basis of densitometric criteria alone. However, for women who are postmenopausal, the WHO definition still seems to hold. Thus, younger women (prior to menopause) are compared to their own age group, while older women are compared (and diagnosed based on that comparison) to healthy twenty-year-olds!

Current treatments focus on bone growth but fail to recognize that remodeling is a balanced process. One of the biggest myths about osteoporosis has to do with calcium. While the dairy industry would have people believe that dietary calcium is critical to bone formation and that the best way to get that calcium is milk products, there is mounting evidence that this is not so. Yes, calcium is an important component of healthy bone, but dairy products may not be the best way to get that calcium. Calcium from milk is in the form of calcium lactate, which is not as easily absorbed as other forms that can be found in green, leafy vegetables. Milk consumption in Greece doubled from 1961 to 1977 (and was even higher in 1985), and from 1977 to 1985 the age-adjusted osteoporosis incidence almost doubled, too.[15] In Hong Kong, twice as much dairy products were consumed in 1989 as compared to 1966, and incidence of osteoporosis tripled in the same period.[16] Americans consume large amounts of dairy products, and thus take in extremely high levels of calcium, but they also sustain high rates of osteoporosis and osteoporosis-related fractures.[17, 18]

While calcium is surely an essential part of bone formation, there is currently no substantial data showing that increased consumption of dairy products prevents or slows down the development of osteoporosis. In fact, according to a 1985 study in the *American Journal of Clinical Nutrition*, the more milk women drank, the more bone loss they experienced.[19] Current recommendations from the Harvard School of Public Health are that women should get calcium as much as possible from green, leafy vegetables rather than from dairy products.[20]

The Osteoporosis Foundation and American Dietetic Association both receive money from the dairy industry. According to the Physicians Committee for Responsible Medicine (PCRM), there is a lack of credible research showing a deficiency in calcium is to blame for current osteoporosis epidemic! In fact, one study tracked eighty-one girls ages twelve to eighteen for six years. Their calcium intake was controlled by supplementation (using calcium supplements rather than foods), and the conclusion was that increased calcium supplementation was not associated with hip bone density at age eighteen or with total body bone mineral gain at ages twelve through eighteen.[21]

According to PCRM people should limit animal protein intake as animal protein leaches calcium from bones. Animal proteins are high in sulfur-containing amino acids (especially cysteine and methionine). When these break down, sulfur is converted to sulfate, which acidifies the blood. More acidic blood dissolves calcium from bone. Additionally, carbonated soft drinks have been implicated in leaching calcium from bone. However, there is proof that some other approaches can help allay bone loss. Weight-bearing exercise is helpful for bone density increase, as is yoga to relieve stress, which can be associated with bone loss. Also, people should limit cigarettes, salt, caffeine, and a sedentary lifestyle.

HORMONES AND BONE HEALTH

As mentioned earlier, bone loss accelerates during menopause. Hormonal changes after menopause increase the rate of bone resorption, leading to a greater risk of osteoporosis. Progesterone builds bone, and the loss of this critical hormone means that new bone is not being synthesized. In a three-year study with postmenopausal women treated with natural progesterone, bone density increased by about 15 percent.[22]

When synthetic hormones first came on the market, they were touted as being great for preventing or slowing the progress of osteoporosis. However, since the WHI study was halted, there have been very few options for women who want to keep healthy bones. This is one of the key benefits of bioidentical hormones for women. A combination of dietary changes (including getting calcium from green, leafy vegetables) as well as regular exercise and supplementation with bioidentical hormones can go a long way toward helping women keep their bones strong. Estrogen, progesterone, and testosterone are all important in supporting the process of bone remodeling.

ALZHEIMER'S AND GENERAL DEMENTIA

I have had clients and friends in their sixties and early seventies diagnosed with Alzheimer's. There seems to be so much more cognitive decline now that one has to wonder: Is this a function of many living longer? Is this a function of environmental impact? There are no simple answers.

According to Julian Whitaker, MD, while much of the information on Alzheimer's prevention and dementia comes from mainstream medical sources, most of it is not being used because it is not patentable; in other words, only drugs that can make money are generally promoted, while nutritional supplements exist such as fish and flax oils that are anti-inflammatory are not generally touted. Yes, there are physicians that will tell their patients to supplement with fish and flax oils, but they are not promoted in the same way as pharmaceuticals. The available drugs used are called cholinesterase inhibitors that block the breakdown of acetylcholine, a neurotransmitter involved in cognitive retention. There is a newer class of drug called memantine HCl that proponents claim works well in conjunction with the more commonly used medications. However, when I searched the literature looking for actual rate or time of cognitive decline improvements, the language was uniformly vague. Unfortunately, while these cholinesterase inhibitors, and more recently dopamine-stimulating drugs, may slow the progress of rapid dementia for perhaps three to six months, that is the best they can do.

Memory loss and the dementia umbrella now have become a huge market for drugs that do little, really. Proponents of these drugs say they delay the advancing symptoms for six to twelve months in 10 to 20 percent of the people who take them—dismal statistics for those promoting a drug to the tune of $1,500 per year. One has to wonder if simple drugs such as aspirin or ibuprofen may do more to curb inflammatory tendencies than these ineffective and expensive cholinesterase inhibitors. While there is an excellent study comparing the use of the most commonly used drugs for dementia and available nutrient biochemicals,[23] more studies need to be done relating diet to Alzheimer's. For instance, a diet high in animal foods is also high in arachidonic acid, which is known to be a proinflammatory molecule. Perhaps a diet that is more plant based could help in terms of dietary impacts. I think medicine is really at an impasse here as many are living longer, and not so well. While doctors are trying hard to find some solutions, most of what is available pharmaceutically is really palliative.

Biochemical researchers have found that degenerative changes in the brain are linked to chronic inflammation that causes toxins to be released, producing a cascade of free radicals that damage brain cells.[24] There are protective nutrients such as certain B vitamins, and methylated forms of B12 and folic acid, that inhibit free radical formation; some of these are similar to drugs that lower homocysteine for better heart function. For years we have worked with 5-MTHF (methylated folic acid). Now a relatively new drug, Deplin, has come out that is based on MTHF and is being marketed as a "medical food" that supposedly can enhance the effectiveness of other mood-altering drugs. We have found certain nutrients, such as 5-MTHF, extremely helpful for enhancing cognition and some aspects of memory. Many nutrients also play a role in reducing free radical damage. These include antioxidant vitamins (notably vitamin C) and various detoxifying amino acids, such as N-acetylcysteine.

There are neuronutrients called "nootropics," such as Piracetam, that are designed to bolster cerebral blood flow between the two brain hemispheres. This is nonaddictive, well tolerated, and available without a prescription.

There are also studies involving herbs such as curcumin that appear to have potent anti-inflammatory potential, and this lessens damage to neurons.[25]

While there has been conflicting information on caffeine, it now appears that small amounts are good for the aging brain for people who are not vulnerable to high anxiety. Caffeine has benefits for short-term cognition and retention, and it also helps protect against neurodegenerative disease. Men who regularly drink coffee are far less likely to develop Parkinson's disease. In the *Journal of Alzheimer's Disease*, those who used caffeine were reported to show significant less progression of memory loss in older people with mild cognitive impairment.[26]

HORMONES AND ALZHEIMER'S

Returning to hormones that are the basis of this book, numerous studies indicate that neurotoxins, such as beta-amyloid, are elevated in Alzheimer's patients, particularly when primary estrogen is low in women and when testosterone is low in men. It appears that relatively small amounts of estrogen (the amount normally present in a healthy woman in her premenopausal days) may inhibit the development of dementia in many forms.

Brain tissue in Alzheimer's patients is full of inflammatory chemicals, and there are biological counters to some inflammatory markers, such as C-reactive protein (CRP); this is often elevated long before neurological symptoms develop.[27] Estrogen enhances blood flow to the brain and inhibits free radical formation. One of the functions is to decrease glutamate excitotoxicity at the NMDA receptors, allowing proper calcium ionic channel function. Further, patients with Alzheimer's and other dementias are often prescribed antidepressants and other drugs to counter symptoms; these further deplete crucial nutrients such as glutathione and CoQ-10. We often give women with memory issues N-acetyl cysteine (NAC) that helps the body absorb glutathione, as it is poorly absorbed when taken orally. NAC improves cognition.[28]

I see a number of women who are not so old—many in their early seventies—who are experiencing more than casual memory loss, and their families are at a loss, often feeling burdened by the simplest routines of being supportive. And when does being supportive turn to complete sacrifice? At what point does one throw in the towel and say he cannot do this anymore? It is far easier to care for someone if there has been great love; far harder if the relationship had been waning for years. But the same questions exist. So often these questions appear unanswerable, but I often steer family members to get to a place of relief—that simple word can make a huge difference. If one is staggering under the enormity of a problem, looking for just a step in the direction of relief is profound. This can be getting psychological support for oneself, if the couple is too far gone, all the way to recognizing that outside help is truly needed, and when to commit to exploring the next level of care.

FINDING BALANCE AS WE AGE

In our rural resort mountain town in Colorado, the summer population swells to more than double that of the off season. Those of us who have remained here year round for many years have seen the aging demographic of this summer crowd. These are the cultural elite, who come for the music and the fine dining and the endless potential to be engaged in one seminar after another. One can avoid facing the issues of aging for a while here.

But still the clock ticks. The average summer resident in Aspen, Colorado, is seventy-five. Many of the women I see became interested in health when it became a cultural statement, about ten to fifteen years ago. I see those who drank like fish and ate tons of red meat now being extreme in how they live and eat; still, genetics and time and gravity will have their way with most. Many are on the diet of the month—they assume whatever is current must be true. For a while, it was Atkins to lose weight (high animal protein, and very unhealthy) or Pritikin (very high carbohydrates). Now many say they are gluten sensitive or cannot eat any dairy. While there are true cases of gluten and lactose intolerance, many of these women are just jumping on the current fad. I find these food sensitivities more prevalent in children who have compromised behavioral and learning skills; indeed, much of this information originally came from the DAN (Defeat Autism Now) conferences, as this population appears to have greater difficulty metabolizing certain proteins (peptides) from foods.

For years, we have highly recommended that most women lean toward a plant- based diet, but some cannot eat this way. However, the women I generally see thriving have cut down in animal food intake. Dairy intake is more toward sheep and goat cheeses, and lots of brassica family (cabbage family: broccoli, cauliflower) vegetables are consumed to modulate good versus less good estrogens.

Depending on the woman a small amount of wine can be beneficial; wine contains great antioxidants such as resveratrol. A powerful antioxidant that supports cardiovascular health, it's also been shown to help support healthy platelet function and maintain healthy arachidonic acid metabolism. It is also relaxing and helps some with social anxiety, again in moderation.

They cannot turn back the clock, however. They may have all the plastic surgery in the world, yet the bones are weakening and the muscles are losing collagen. Bioidentical hormones can be a great support, emotionally as well as physically.

Last week, I saw a seventy-six-year-old woman who is so determined to stay forever young that it must be unconsciously exhausting to keep pushing the rock uphill. I do not know how I will feel at that age, assuming I make it, but I hope to have an element of acceptance through each passage in my life and still look and feel as well as I can.

And yet, for this woman, a modest dose of bioidentical hormones would go a long way to bolstering her self-confidence and removing some of the obstacles associated with not being young and sexy forever. This perception of needing to be static in time is a problem with much of the anti-aging discourse today. There is a quality of exhaustion to the constant striving—the need for always thinking one is alpha.

From repeated conversations with women from all over who have come here to see me and the doctors I have worked with around the country, I know this to be a fact: intelligent, grounded women are living in the present, in their bodies now. They are not looking to be ferociously or obviously sexy as their first draw. They certainly want to be sexual and deeply compelling and attractive to their partners. Finding balance and rational happiness is the answer, I think, in any generation for all time. The essential nature of human happiness does not change generation to generation.

ATTITUDE

I see it with the women and the men, in different ways. Joseph Campbell, in his book *This Business of the Gods*,[29] talks about how at his age—then nearing eighty—it must become a time for reflection, of not of striving any longer. So how is one to have an optimal quality to these years of midlife and beyond? Perhaps it needs to begin with acceptance of the journey and recognition that one cannot control everything. But one can be a vital, creative force in one's own life at any age or stage.

There is another marvelous book, a classic written in 1988 titled *Who Gets Sick* by Blair Justice, PhD. He talks about the need for autonomy in order to get past catastrophe, or trauma, or just the difficulties of living.[30] The premise of Dr. Justice's book is that the more autonomy one has over one's thinking and sense of life, the more we can persevere when life truly seems to spiral down, out of our control.

Robert Johnson, in his book *Living Your Unlived Life*,[31] talks about finding the other sides of happiness that have eluded one in the first half or two-thirds of life: he asks, How do we bring to consciousness those unlived parts of our selves? First, someone has to want to. For most, it is easier to avoid going deeper at a time when one may be yearning for peace. Often, for a life capable of great depth there requires a descent of staggering proportions. Often this follows death of a great love, an illness from which recovery is happening, divorce, or some other unexpected major life event. This often allows the psyche to plunge into the unknown depths that were invisible before.

Our hormones plunge as our psyches descend. This is, of course, because high stress depletes all the gender hormones; and again, as cortisol, the stress hormone rises, DHEA, the key anti-aging molecule, descends. This is the dance of the molecules, and where the knowledge we teach women, from years of research, is so valuable. I also work with the feeling state of women and teach them to bring forth the way they wish to feel about any given subject and to align themselves with that in their thoughts and conversations. This takes us to a sense of manifesting the best possible outcome. Life can be very challenging even for the strongest person; in fact, people become strong through trial by fire.

DESCENTS AND ASCENTS: THE CYCLES OF LIFE

In the preface to this book, I described my own terrible descent into the sadness of life with my husband's illness and death. When he finally told me I had to let him go, I felt as if the world stopped. And indeed it has seemed to for the past three years. I have only recently felt a true sense of renewal about my future. I have a lot of hope for our son.

During this time, I have witnessed the plummeting of my own hormone levels, and I have used myself to further test a working hypothesis (with women I have tracked over the years) that when women are going through extreme stress they need more hormones, not less.[32]

I have seen greatly reduced primary estrogen levels in blood tests repeatedly in others going through trauma and in myself. In my single case, I have tracked many lab samples and correlated them with mood changes, and the data is startling. When I see the lowest E2 (estradiol) levels at a time when I am using higher amounts of estrogen than usual, this is startling. My brain and nervous system are "soaking it up." Other women in long-term observation have reported similar effects, working with me and with various physicians around the country. While we are always teaching women to monitor the usually obvious signs of rare estrogen excess, more often we see low levels of estrogen with very stressful life situations. When things resolve the need lessens.

Despite all the despair of the last three years, my capacity for happiness still exists—why is it that those with a truly great capacity for joy often are put to the test? I have been tested in major ways in my life, both personally, with the illness of my husband, and in my work, where I have found that many traditionally trained doctors are afraid to even look at the research and listen to the information that I have about bioidentical hormones. While both of these experiences have made me disillusioned with the state of the medical establishment, I know that there are some great physicians out there, and there are many people ready to listen to new discourses about emotional wellness. This book is an attempt to reach those people and to open up some new conversations for women so that they can age with grace and power.

APPENDIX: HOW TO USE BIOIDENTICAL HORMONES

Below is a guide to the use of bioidentical hormones. Of course, you the reader must work with the best health care professional you can find to get the help you need, and each person is responsible for her own well-being. The following are recommendations and are not intended as advice for specific individuals.

WHICH HORMONE TO USE FIRST?

I always get blood levels prior to starting someone on bioidentical hormones. Once I have those initial levels, I rely on patient symptoms to guide me. Very often, I use several different hormones in combination (compounded into a single cream), but for the sake of simplicity for the reader, I have broken this chapter into sections for the different hormones individually.

PROGESTERONE

Even if a woman has had a hysterectomy, she still needs progesterone. There are progesterone receptors in the brain; behind the eye in the entire nasal pharyngeal passages; in the joints; and can be taken as a neurosteroid; it may be involved in many more neuromodulating functions that we are not yet aware of.

As mentioned throughout this book, I only use bioidentical progesterone, which is the exact molecule that your body produces. This is often derived from the soybean plant. While it may be *synthesized* in a laboratory, it is not a *synthetic* product.

Premenstrual Syndrome (PMS)

Bioidentical progesterone is the molecule of choice for many mood and other symptoms of PMS, and it is crucial for anxiety, whether or not a woman has a uterus.

What are the symptoms?

1. Mood swings
2. Fluid retention
3. Fibroids or cysts
4. Short cycles
5. High levels of stress

For cycling women:
Do you know when you ovulate?

1. Begin taking progesterone at the time of ovulation.
2. Continue until you know the symptoms are gone, even if it means completely throughout your period. If the symptoms cease with the beginning of flow, stop then.

I usually have menstruating women use progesterone until her period starts, but if mood symptoms are persistent, or cramping occurs, then keep using it.

Dosage:

1. The average dose should be 400 mg per day—100 mg taken at breakfast, lunch, dinner, and bedtime.
2. A woman can take up to 800 mg per day.
3. Do not take 200 mg at one time. This could lead to extreme drowsiness. It would be appropriate to use at bedtime, however.

Infertility (Luteal Phase Defect)

Dosage:

1. Begin dosage at ovulation of 400 mg per day (best to check between 10 a.m. and 12 noon). This should produce levels as high as 25 ng/ml. Do not hesitate to take 800 mg per day, if necessary.
2. It is still being argued today that progesterone cannot be taken orally. Goodman and Gilman state that progesterone is rapidly destroyed through portal excretion to the liver. The real culprit is stomach acid. When the progesterone is suspended in oil, it becomes a fat, and 90 percent of all fats taken into the body are picked up through the lymphatic system. Progesterone prepared in this manner (as a suspension in oil) will produce consistent and quality blood levels.
3. I prefer transdermal hormones in most cases: the upper GI metabolites formed from oral progesterone make some women more down and depressed, particularly those already vulnerable to depression. The only time I use oral progesterone is for insomnia in women not prone to depression.

Menopause

Progesterone is used here to oppose or balance estrogen, particularly to protect the uterus. However, progesterone levels usually decline well before menopause, and progesterone can have a very calming effect at this time. This can happen in a wide range of ages, and it doesn't have to fit the model of fifty-one-and-a-half years.

Dosage:
Usual starting dose is 200 mg per day, 100 mg taken twice daily.

Osteoporosis

Progesterone acts on the osteoblast receptors to increase bone synthesis. Estrogen acts on the osteoclasts to slow bone-mass breakdown. Progesterone not only helps to prevent osteoporosis but also will reverse it. Our experience has been that the worse the condition, the faster the reversal.

Dosage:
    200 mg to 400 mg per day, taken twice daily.

ESTROGEN

This is the exact molecule produced by the body. Like progesterone, it may be derived from soybean plants. There are three main types:

1. Estrone—commonly referred to as E1; it is twelve times weaker than estradiol and is produced from estradiol in the stomach and liver.
2. Estradiol—commonly referred to as E2; it is the most potent form of estrogen and the main estrogen produced by the ovaries.
3. Estriol—commonly referred to as E3; it is the weakest form, eighty times weaker than estradiol, and it is produced by the conversion of estrone in the liver.

Even though estriol is the weakest form of estrogen, it appears to be an important form, as it addresses the vagina, the uterus, and the bladder. It is vital for lubrication. The best method for giving estriol for these reasons—vaginal dryness, prolapsed uterus, lack of bladder muscle tone—is to use a vaginal cream, which contains 0.6 mg/gm of cream. The dosage most commonly prescribed is to insert 1 gram vaginally at bedtime for one week, then as needed, one to three times per week.

Estradiol was getting a "bad rap" after the Women's Health Initiative (WHI) Study. Based on much research, I, and many medical colleagues, firmly believe that if estradiol is properly opposed with progesterone, it is not the "bad guy." Estradiol is known to be important in muscle integrity. Estradiol has given women a definite cardiovascular advantage over men, working through lipoprotein synthesis, fatty acid metabolism, as well as muscle integrity. Estradiol exerts activity on the epithelial tissue as well. This is shown in "hot flash" research (e.g., if a women is connected to a monitor, it is possible to detect a "hot flash" seventeen seconds before it is felt by the patient). This is the critical estrogen for containing the rusting (oxidative stress) of aging, and it is so vital for cognitive function.

Dosage:

1. Usual starting dosage is 0.5 mg twice daily. This can be given separately or compounded in the same capsule with 100 mg bio-identical progesterone.
2. Some women need more (many menopausal women report needing at least 1 to 1.5 mg in the morning and 0.5 to 1.5 in the evening). This is fine if there are no signs of excess—the most obvious is breast tenderness. This can be safely done *under a physician's guidance.*
3. A woman who has been without hormone replacement for years should probably start with a dosage of estradiol 0.25 mg and progesterone 50 mg twice daily. This dose may be increased until symptoms subside or breast tenderness occurs.
4. We often find that many women need more E2 to feel optimal, and we increase progesterone accordingly, for balance.
5. Dr. Bronson's recent data suggest that when there is trauma, extreme stress, deep sadness, or post-traumatic stress disorder (PTSD), the tissue demand for hormones dramatically increases as indicated by laboratory blood levels.

TESTOSTERONE

This is an androgen (male hormone) that is, like all hormones, involved in many systems throughout the body. We use a bioidentical form (produced from soybeans), which is an exact duplicate of the molecule our body produces. It is the sexual hormone of the male; however, it is vital for females, though in far lesser amounts. It is responsible for many of the same positive hormonal responses as estrogen has in females, such as muscle integrity; giving strength, energy, and stamina; and self-esteem.

Most traditional laboratory ranges that I see will indicate that a testosterone level of less than 30 ng/dL is normal. Based on my work I assert that a "normal" laboratory value of testosterone in women should be between 50 to 80 ng/dL. Telling women that a level of less than 30 ng/dL is good is analogous to telling someone they have enough vitamin C not to have scurvy, but not enough to prevent the flu or to enhance immune function.

Lack of testosterone may be involved in connective tissue disorders. Lupus occurs five times more often in females than in males. According to Dr. Jonathan Wright, he has never seen a case of lupus in which the testosterone level was above 20 ng/dL. This has been my experience now in literally dozens of cases and with every physician that I have shared this information with.

For men reading . . .

The normal level for males in their prime (twenty-one years of age) is 1,000 to 1,200 ng/dL. Men lose about 50 percent of their testosterone from age twenty-five to fifty. The percentage drop is more critical than the actual numerical values. This drop is most noticeable for men when the decrease is a large percentage from the starting point. For example, if the highest levels were 600 and they are now at 400, it is not as serious as if the highest was 1,000 and is now less than 500.

DHEA

This is a neurosteroid produced in the nervous system. I use a plant-derived bioidentical form synthesized from the root of the Barbosco plant. It is often referred to in the literature as a *mother hormone*.

Indications:

Dr. William Regelson, who probably has done more research on DHEA than anyone else, claims that DHEA has many indications and functions as everything from an immune system modulator to a blood sugar balancer. In his book *DHEA: The Super Hormone*, he states that the key seems to be in restoring DHEA levels to the levels of your youth. He claims that the youthful serum levels are 400 to 560 mcg/dL of blood for men and 350 to 430 mcg/dL for women. Immune system support is probably the most common prescription use that I see. The feedback from patients most commonly heard is an increase in energy, strength, and stamina. This probably can help explain the positive response from many chronic fatigue patients.

Dosage:

1. For males: 50 to 100 mg per day.
2. For females: 15 to 25 mg per day.
3. We recommend starting women at 5 mg per day, increasing at intervals of 2.5 mg as needed for energy and cortisol (stress hormone) reduction.
4. Some women are so sensitive that they cannot exceed 5 mgs per day; this is fairly rare, but DHEA can make them feel jittery, as if they had consumed a lot of caffeine. If so, the dosage can simply be reduced or stopped and can be countered with additional progesterone.
5. Most women are fine on 5 to 10 mg; the higher doses recommended in certain health magazines seem excessive to us based on the serious literature: the goal is balance.

REFERENCES

Baulieu, E., and P. Robel. 1998, April. Dehydroepiandrosterone (DHEA) and Dehydroepiandrosterone Sulfate (DHEAS) as neuroactive neurosteroids. *Proceedings of the National Academy of Sciences* 95:4089–91.

Check, J. H., MD, and H. G. Adelson. 1987, March–April. The efficacy of progesterone in achieving successful pregnancy: II. In women with pure luteal phase defects. *International Journal of Fertility* 32, no. 2:139–41.

Dalton, K., MD, with W. Holton. 1999. *Once a month: Understanding and treating PMS.* Alameda, CA: Hunter House, Inc.

Gaby, A., MD. 1996. Dehydroepiandrosterone: Biological effects and clinical significance. *Alternative Medicine Review* 1, no. 2:60–69.

———. 1994. Estrogen replacement therapy. In *Preventing & reversing osteoporosis.* New York: Three Rivers Press.

Hargrove, J. T., MD, W. S. Maxson, MD, and A. Colston Wentz, MD. 1989, October. Absorption of oral progesterone is influenced by vehicle and particle size. *American Journal of Obstetrics and Gynecology* 161, no. 4:948–51.

Hargrove, J. T., MD, W. S. Maxson, MD, A. Colston Wentz, MD, and L. S. Burnett, MD. 1989, April. Menopausal hormone replacement therapy with continuous daily oral micronized estradiol and progesterone. *Obstetrics and Gynecology* 73, no. 4:606–12.

Hargrove, J. T., MD, and K. G. Osteen, PhD. 1995, October. An alternative method of hormone replacement therapy using the natural sex steroids. *Infertility and Reproductive Medicine Clinics of North America* 6, no. 4:653–74.

Head, K. A., ND. 1998. Estriol: Safety and efficacy. *Alternative Medicine Review* 3, no. 2:101–13.

Kalimi, M., and W. Regelson. 1990. *The biologic role of Dehydroepiandrosterone (DHEA).* Boston: Walter de Gruyter Publishing, 361–85.

Mooradian, A. D., J. E. Morley, and S. G. Korenman. 1987, February. Biological actions of androgens. *Endocrine Society* 8, no. 1:1–28.

Prior, J. C., MD. 1990, May. Progesterone as a bone-trophic hormone. *Endocrine Reviews* 11, no. 2:386–98.

Prior, J. C., MD, Y. Vigna, RN, and N. Alojado, RN. 1991. Progesterone and the prevention of osteoporosis. *Canadian Journal of Obstetrics/Gynecology and Women's Health Care* 3, no. 4:178–84.

Raz, R., MD, and W. E. Stamm, MD. 1993, September. A controlled trial of intravaginal estriol in postmenopausal women with recurrent urinary tract infections. *New England Journal of Medicine* 329, no. 11:753–56.

Regelson, William, and Carol Colman. 1997. *The Superhormone Promise*. New York: Pocket Books.

Rosick, E. R., DO, MPH, MS. 2004, April. Why aging women need testosterone. *Life Extension Magazine*:53–59.

Tenover, J. S. 1992, October. Effects of testosterone supplementation in the aging male. *Journal of Clinical Endocrinology and Metabolism* 75, no. 4:1092–98.

Winters, S. J., MD. 1999, May–June. Current status of testosterone replacement therapy in men. *Clinical Review*.

Wright, J. V., MD, B. Schliesman, MCT, and L. Robinson, MCT. 1999. Comparative measurements of serum estriol, estradiol, and estrone in non-pregnant, premenopausal women: A preliminary investigation. *Alternative Medicine Review* 4, no. 4:266–70.

NOTES

INTRODUCTION: WOMEN AND THEIR MOODS

1. K. Miyagawa, J. Rösch, F. Stanczyk, and K. Hermsmeyer, "Medroxypro-gesterone Interferes with Ovarian Steroid Protection against Coronary Vasos-pasm," *Nature Medicine* 3, no. 3 (1997): 324–27.

2. Louann Brizendine, *The Female Brain* (New York: Morgan Road/Broadway Books, 2006).

3. N. L. Rasgon, *The Effects of Estrogen on Brain Function* (Baltimore: Johns Hopkins University Press, 2006), 2–3.

1. IN DEFENSE OF ESTROGEN

1. Phyllis Bronson, PhD, "In Defense of Estrogen," *Journal of Orthomo-lecular Medicine* 22, no. 3 (2007).

2. Jeffrey Dach, *Bioidentical Hormones 101* (Davie, FL: Dach Press, 2012), chapter 11.

3. Dach, *Bioidentical Hormones 101.*

4. "FDA Bans Hormone Produced by Human Body as 'Unapproved' Drug," MenopauseGoddessBlog,com, http://www.menopausegoddessblog.com/wp-content/uploads/2008/02/homecoalition_ad.pdf.

5. "FDA Bans Hormone Produced by Human Body as 'Unapproved' Drug."

6. "FDA Bans Hormone Produced by Human Body as 'Unapproved' Drug."

7. Jonathan Wright, "Bolster Your Memory," *Nutrition and Healing* 19, no. 6 (2012).

2. THE TRUTH ABOUT PROGESTERONE

1. John Lee, *What Your Doctor May Not Tell You about Breast Cancer* (New York: Warner Books, 2002), 149.

2. Kent Holtorf, MD, "The Bioidentical Hormone Debate: Are Bioidentical Hormones (Estradiol, Estriol, and Progesterone) Safer or More Efficacious Than Commonly Used Synthetic Versions in Hormone Replacement Therapy?" *Postgraduate Medicine* 121, no. 1 (January 2009), http://jeffreydach.com/files/80618-70584/The_Bioidentical_Hormone_Debate_Ken_Holtorf_MD.pdf.

3. A. Fournier, F. Berrino, E. Riboli, V. Avenel, and F. Clavel-Chapelon, "Breast Cancer Risks in Relation to Different Types of Hormone Replacement Therapy in the E3N-EPIC Cohort," *International Journal of Cancer* 114, no. 3 (April 2005): 448–54.

4. Jeffrey Dach, *Bioidentical Hormones 101* (Davie, FL: Dach Press, 2012).

5. Erika Schwartz, Kent Holtorf, and David Brownstein, "The Truth about Hormone Therapy," *Wall Street Journal*, March 16, 2009, http://online.wsj.com/article/SB123717056802137143.html.

6. K. Miyagawa and Keith Hermsmeyer, "Medroxyprogesterone Interferes with Ovarian Steroid Protection against Coronary Vasospasm," *Nature Medicine* 3 (March 1997): 324.

7. Holtorf, "The Bioidentical Hormone Debate."

8. Uzzi Reiss, *Natural Hormone Balance for Women* (New York: Pocket Books, 2001), 71, 85.

9. Ryoko Hiroi and John F. Neumaier, "Estrogen Decreases 5-HT$_{1B}$ Autoreceptor mRNA in Selective Subregion of Rat Dorsal Raphe Nucleus: Inverse Association between Gene Expression and Anxiety Behavior in the Open Field," *Neuroscience* 158, no. 2 (January 2009): 456–64, http://www.ncbi.nlm.nih.gov/pmc/articles/PMC2667128/.

10. K. Hermsmeyer and Miyagawa et al., "Reactivity-Based Coronary Vasospasm Independent of Atherosclerosis in Rhesus Monkeys," *Journal of the American College of Cardiology* 29, no. 3 (March 1997): 671.

11. The Writing Group for the PEPI Trial, "Effects of Estrogen or Estrogen/Progestin Regimens on Heart Disease Risk Factors in Postmenopausal Women. The Postmenopausal Estrogen/Progestin Interventions Trial," *Journal of the American Medical Association* 273, no. 3 (1995): 199–208.

12. Writing Group for the PEPI Trial, "Effects of Estrogen or Estrogen/Progestin Regimens."

13. Marion Woodman, *Addiction to Perfection: The Still Unravished Bride* (Toronto: Inner City Books, 1982).

14. "A Lifetime of Progesterone," *Women's Health Connection*, February 2012, http://www.womensinternational.com/pdf/progesterone.pdf.

15. Alan E. Beer, MD, "Progesterone Levels during Pregnancy," Finch University of Health Science, Chicago Medical School, Chicago, Illinois, 2001.

16. "A Lifetime of Progesterone."

17. "A Lifetime of Progesterone."

18. "A Lifetime of Progesterone."

19. Helen Saul Case, *The Vitamin Cure for Women's Health Problems*, Vitamin Cure Series (Laguna Beach, CA: Basic Health, 2012).

20. Abram Hoffer, *Adventures in Psychiatry* (Toronto: KOS Publishing, 2005).

21. Women's Health Connection online interview, February 2012. https://65.119.211.170/owa/redir.aspx?C=39d871adbb994d51b6d4700109b8605b&URL=http%3a%2f%2fwww.womensinternational.com%2fnewsletter%2farticl e_bronson.html%3futm_source%3dMarch%2b2012%2bNewsletter%26utm_c ampaign%3dFeb%2b2012%2bNewsletter%26utm_medium%3demail.

3. MOOD CHEMISTRY

1. Phyllis Bronson, "A Biochemist's Experience with GABA," *Journal of Orthomolecular Medicine* 26, no. 1 (2011).

2. Marcia Angell, "The Illusions of Psychiatry," *New York Times* Book Review, July 14, 2011.

3. John Oldman, Daniel Carlat, Richard Friedman, and Andrew Nierenberg, reply by Marcia Angell, "'The Illusions of Psychiatry': An Exchange," New York Review of Books, August 18, 2011.

4. Mark Zimmerman, *Interview Guide for Evaluating DSM-IV Psychiatric Disorders and the Mental Status Examination* (East Greenwich, RI: Psychiatric Products Press, 1994), 40.

5. Peter Breggin, *Toxic Psychiatry* (New York: St. Martin's Press, 1991), 324.

6. Andrius Baskys and Gary Remington, *Brain Mechanisms and Psychotropic Drugs* (New York: CRC Press, 1996), 56–58.

7. Peter D. Kramer, *Listening to Prozac* (New York: Penguin Books, 1997).

8. Peter Breggin, *Talking Back to Prozac* (New York: St. Martin's Paperbacks, 1995).

9. Peter Breggin, *Medication Madness* (New York: St. Martin's Press, 2008).

10. Jeffrey Dach, *Bioidentical Hormones 101* (Davie, FL: Dach Press, 2012).

11. Edward Klaiber, *Hormones and the Mind* (New York: Harper Paperbacks, 2002), 161.

12. Daniel DeNoon, "Sleeping Pills Called 'as Risky as Cigarettes,'" WebMD Health News, http://www.webmd.com/sleep-disorders/news/20120227/sleeping-pills-called-as-risky-as-cigarettes.

13. David Gutierrez, "Antidepressant Drugs Linked to School Shootings," NaturalNews.com, April 2, 2008, http://www.naturalnews.com/022930_drugs_antidepressant_drug.html.

14. Bronson, "A Biochemist's Experience with GABA."

15. Zimmerman, *Interview Guide for Evaluating DSM-IV Psychiatric Disorders*, 40.

16. Herschel Sidransky, *Tryptophan: Biochemical and Health Implications* (New York: CRC Press, 2002), 227, 242.

17. Sidransky, *Tryptophan*.

18. Sidransky, *Tryptophan*.

19. Sidransky, *Tryptophan*.

20. Sheryl S. Smith, *Neurosteroid Effects in the Central Nervous System: The Role of the GABA-A Receptor* (Boca Raton, FL: CRC Press, 2003), 174.

21. Smith, *Neurosteroid Effects in the Central Nervous System*.

22. Eric Braverman, *The Edge Effect* (New York: Sterling Publishing, 2004).

23. Abram Hoffer, *Adventures in Psychiatry* (Canada: KOS Publishing, 2005), 42, 200.

4. THE CONNECTION BETWEEN BODY TYPE AND HORMONES

1. Uzzi Reiss, *Natural Hormone Balance for Women* (New York: Pocket Books, 2001), 31–36.

2. Elizabeth Lee Vliet, *It's My Ovaries, Stupid!* (New York: Scribner, 2003), 16–19.

3. Phyllis J. Bronson, "Mood Biochemistry of Women at Mid-Life," *Journal of Orthomolecular Medicine* 16, no. 3 (2001): 141.

4. Candace Pert, *Molecules of Emotion: The Science behind Mind-Body Medicine* (New York: Scribner, 2007), 299.

5. Phyllis J. Bronson, "A Biochemist's Experience with GABA-A Receptor," *Journal of Orthomolecular Medicine* 26, no. 1 (2011).

6. Bronson, "A Biochemist's Experience with GABA-A Receptor."

7. Vliet, *It's My Ovaries, Stupid!*

8. Bronson, "A Biochemist's Experience with GABA-A Receptor."

9. Reiss, *Natural Hormone Balance for Women*, 31–36.

10. Jeffrey Dach, MD, *Bioidentical Hormones 101* (Davie, FL: Dach Press, 2012).

5. WEAVING THE WEB: HOW HORMONES ARE CENTRAL TO THE FEMALE PSYCHE

1. Phyllis Bronson, "The Mood Biochemistry of Women at Mid-Life," *Journal of Orthomolecular Medicine* 16, no. 3 (2001).

2. "Headaches and Hormones," *Women's Health Connection* 9, no. 3 (2010).

3. A. J. Gelenberg, J. D. Wojcik, and W. E. Falk et al., "Tyrosine for Depression: A Double-Blind Trial," *Journal of Affective Disorders* 19 (1990): 125–32.

4. Carolyn Myss, *Why People Don't Heal and How They Can* (New York: Harmony Books, 1997).

5. Sheryl S. Smith, *Neurosteroid Effects in the Central Nervous System: The Role of the GABA-A Receptor* (Boca Raton: CRC Press, 2003), 63.

6. "Chronic Inflammation: "The Silent Enemy Burning Within," *Connections*, WomensInternational.com, 2012, http://www.womensinternational.com/pdf/Inflammation.pdf.

7. "Chronic Inflammation: "The Silent Enemy Burning Within."

8. Michael Meade, *The Water of Life: Initiation and Tempering of the Soul* (Seattle: Greenfire Press Mosaic Foundation, 2006), 86, 88; Michael Meade, *The World behind the World* (Seattle: Greenfire Press Mosaic Foundation, 2006).

6. SEXUALITY

1. Andy Newman, "What Women Want (Maybe)," NewYorkTimes.com, June 12, 2008, http://www.nytimes.com/2008/06/12/fashion/12bisex.html?pagewanted=all&_r=0.

2. Steven Hotze, *Hormones, Health, and Happiness* (Houston: Forrest Publishing, 2005), 119.

3. Christiane Northrup, *The Wisdom of Menopause* (New York: Bantam Books, 2001), 251.

4. Northrup, *The Wisdom of Menopause*, 251.

5. M. Wafaa, Aboul Enien, Nadia A. Barghash, and Fayrouz S. Mohamed Ali, "Clinical, Ultrasonographic and Endocrine Predictors of Ovarian Response to Clomiphene Citrate in Normogonadotropic Anovulatory Infertility," *Middle East Fertility Society Journal* 3, no. 9 (2006): 242–50.

6. Eugene Shippen, *The Testosterone Syndrome* (New York: M. Evans and Co., 1998).

7. Louise Hay, *You Can Heal Your Life* (Carlsbad, CA: Hay House, 1984).

8. Richard Lord, B. Bongiovanni, and J. A. Bralley, "Estrogen Metabolism and the Diet-Cancer Connection: Rationale for Assessing the Ratio of Urinary Hydroxylated Estrogen Metabolites," *Alternative Medicine Review* 7, no. 2 (2002).

9. Women's Health Connection is from the educational arm of Women's International Pharmacy. Past e-newsletters are available from: http://www.womensinternational.com/newsletter/index.html, and they offer the *Connections* newsletter online as well: http://www.womensinternational.com/connections/index.html.

10. *Women's Health Connection*, DHEA, Wisconsin (May 2012).

11. Elizabeth Lee Vliet, *The Savvy Woman's Guide to Testosterone* (Tucson: Her Place Press, 2005).

12. Joyce Carol Oates, *A Widow's Story* (New York: Ecco/Harper Collins), 2011.

7. EMOTIONS AND RELATIONSHIPS

1. John Bradshaw, *Healing the Shame That Binds You* (Deerfield Beach, FL: Recovery Classics, 2005).

2. Debra Tannen, *You Just Don't Understand* (New York: HarperCollins, 1990).

3. John Gray, *Men Are from Mars, Women Are from Venus* (New York: HarperCollins, 2004).

4. Patricia Evans, *The Verbally Abusive Relationship* (Avon, MA: Adams Media, 2000).

5. Uzzi Reiss, *Natural Hormone Balance* (New York: Pocket Books, 2001), 34.

6. Robert Johnson, *He, She, and We* (trilogy) (New York: Harper Perennial, 1989 and WE HarperOne, 1985).

7. Robert Moore, *King, Warrior, Magician, Lover* (New York: HarperOne, 1991).

8. Linda Schierse Leonard, *The Wounded Woman* (Boston: Shambala, 1998).

8. DISEASES OF AGING/ADVENTURES IN AGING

1. Siddhartha Mukerjee, *The Emperor of All Maladies* (New York: Scribner, 2011).

2. Samuel Epstein, *The Politics of Cancer* (New York: East Ridge Press, 1998).

3. Julian Whitaker, "Thirty Years of Saving Lives," *Townsend Letter* (August/ September 2008): 75.

4. Christiane Northrup, "Breast Health," *Christiane Northrup Newsletter* 4, no. 12 (December 1997).

5. Jeffrey Dach, MD, *Bioidentical Hormones 101* (Davie, FL: Dach Press, 2012).

6. Dach, *Bioidentical Hormones 101*.

7. Dach, *Bioidentical Hormones 101*.

8. Suzanne Somers, "Hormones . . . the Backbone of Health and Quality of Life," written interview with Jonathan Wright, *The Townsend Letter* (August 2010): 54–63.

9. Kent Holtorf, MD, "The Bioidentical Hormone Debate: Are Bioidentical Hormones (Estradiol, Estriol, and Progesterone) Safer or More Efficacious Than Commonly Used Synthetic Versions in Hormone Replacement Therapy?" *Postgraduate Medicine* 121, no. 1 (January 2009), http://jeffreydach.com/files/80618-70584/The_Bioidentical_Hormone_Debate_Ken_Holtorf_MD.pdf.

10. Somers, "Hormones . . . the Backbone of Health and Quality of Life."

11. Julian Whitaker, "Heart Surgery: Look Before You Leap," *Health and Healing* 22, no. 12 (2012).

12. Jon Kabat-Zinn, *Full Catastrophy Living* (London, UK: Delta Books, 1990).

13. Gillian Sanson, *The Myth of Osteoporosis: What Every Woman Should Know about Creating Bone Health* (MI: MCD Century Publications, 2003).

14. Alan R. Gaby, *Preventing and Reversing Osteoporosis: Every Woman's Essential Guide* (Rocklin, CA: Prima Publishing, 1994).

15. I. Paspati, A. Galanos, and G. P. Lyritis, "Hip Fracture Epidemiology in Greece during 1977–1992," *Calcified Tissue International* 62, no. 6 (June 1998): 542–47.

16. E. M. Lau and C. Cooper, "Epidemiology and Prevention of Osteoporosis in Urbanized Asian Populations," *Osteoporosis* 3, suppl. 1 (1993): 23–26.

17. W. Owusu, W. C. Willett, D. Feskanich, A. Ascherio, D. Spiegelman, and G. A. Colditz, "Calcium Intake and the Incidence of Forearm and Hip Fractures among Men." *Journal of Nutrition* 127, no. 9 (1997): 1782–87.

18. D. Feskanich, W. C. Willett, M. J. Stampfer, and G. A. Colditz, "Milk, Dietary Calcium, and Bone Fractures in Women: A 12-Year Prospective Study," *American Journal of Public Health* 87, no. 6 (1997): 992–97.

19. R. R. Recker and R. P. Heaney, "The Effect of Milk Supplements on Calcium Metabolism, Bone Metabolism and Calcium Balance," *American Journal of Clinical Nutrition* 41, no. 2 (February 1985): 254.

20. See http://www.hsph.harvard.edu/nutritionsource/healthy-eating-plate/.

21. T. Lloyd et al., "Adult Female Hip Bone Density Reflects Teenage Sports-Exercise Patterns but Not Teenage Calcium Intake," *Pediatrics* 106, no. 1 (July 2000): 40–44.

22. J. R. Lee, MD, "Osteoporosis Reversal: The Role of Progesterone," *International Clinical Nutrition Review* 10, no. 3 (July 1990): 384–91.

23. M. Tsolaki, T. Pantazi, and A. Kazis. "Efficacy of Acetylcholinesterase Inhibitors versus Nootropics in Alzheimer's Disease," *Journal of International Medical Research* 29, no. 1 (January–February 2001): 28–36.

24. B. Hooshmand et al., "Association between Serum Homocysteine, Holotranscobalamin, Folate and Cognition in the Elderly: A Longitudinal Study," *Journal of Internal Medicine* 271, no. 2 (February 2012): 204–21.

25. J. Wright, "Bolster Your Memory," *Nutrition and Healing* 19, no. 6 (2012).

26. C. Cao et al., "High Blood Caffeine Levels in MCI Linked to Lack of Progression in Dementia," *Journal of Alzheimer's Disease* 30, no. 3 (2012): 559–72.

27. A. R. Genazzani, *Hormone Replacement Therapy and the Brain* (London: Parthenon, 2003), 14.

28. R. S. Lord, and J. A. Bralley, *Laboratory Evaluations for Integrative and Functional Medicine* (Duluth, GA: Metametrix Institute, 2008).

29. Joseph Campbell, *This Business of the Gods* (Ontario: Canada Windrose Films, 1989).

30. Blair Justice, *Who Gets Sick* (Los Angeles, CA: Tarcher, 1987), 58.

31. Robert A. Johnson, *Living Your Unlived Life* (New York: Tarcher/Penguin, 2007).

32. Karen J. Miller and Steven Rogers, *The Estrogen-Depression Connection: The Hidden Link between Hormones and Women's Depression* (Oakland, CA: New Harbinger 2007), 84.

BIBLIOGRAPHY

GENERAL REFERENCES FOR HORMONE/MOOD ARTICLES AND ABSTRACTS

Adlercreutz, H. "Phytoestrogens: Epidemiology and a Possible Role in Cancer Protection." *Environmental Health Perspective* 103, no. 7 (1995): 103–11, 193.

Amen, Daniel. *Making a Good Brain Great*. New York: Harmony Books, 2005.

Anekwe, Tobenna D. "Profits and Plagiarism: The Case of Medical Ghostwriting." *Bioethics* 24, no. 6 (July 2010): 267–72.

Beer, Alan E., MD. "Progesterone Levels during Pregnancy," Finch University of Health Science, Chicago Medical School, Chicago, Illinois, 2001.

Biegen, Anat. *Sites of Drug Action in the Human Brain*. Boca Raton, FL: CRC Press, 1995.

Bohlen und Halbach, O. von, and R. Dermietzel. *Neurotransmitters and Neuromodulators: Handbook of Receptors and Biological Effects*. Hoboken: Wiley-VCH, 2006.

Boomsma, D. "A Review of Current Research on the Effects of Progesterone." *International Journal of Pharmaceutical Compounding* 6, no. 4 (2002).

Bradlow, H. L., D. W. Sepkovic, N. T. Telang, and M. P. Osborne. "Indole-3-carbinol: A Novel Approach to Breast Cancer Prevention." *Annals of the New York Academy of Science* 768 (1995): 180–200.

Bradlow, H. L., N. T. Telang, D. W. Sepkovic, and M. P. Osborne. "2-hydroxyestrone: The 'Good' Estrogen." *Journal of Endocrinology* 150 (1996): S259–S265.

Braverman, Eric. *The Edge Effect*. New York: Sterling, 2004.

Breggin, Peter. *Toxic Psychiatry*. New York: St. Martin's Press, 1991.

Bronson, P. J. "The Effects of Neurosteroids on Depression in Peri-Menopausal Women." *Journal of Orthomolecular Medicine* 20, no. 3 (2005): 210–13.

———. International Society of Orthomolecular Medicine. 2007 Annual Symposium, Toronto, Ontario, Canada.

———. "Mood Biochemistry of Women at Mid-Life." *Journal of Orthomolecular Medicine* 16, no. 3 (2001): 141–54.

Cekic, M., and Donald Stein. "Progesterone Treatment for Brain Injury: An Update," *Future Neurology* 5, no. 1 (2010): 37–46.

Chan, E. K., D. W. Sepkovic, H. J. Yoo Bowne, G. P. Yu, and S. P. Schantz. "A Hormonal Association between Estrogen Metabolism and Proliferative Thyroid Disease." *Otolaryngology–Head and Neck Surgery* 134 (2006): 893–900.

Check, J. H., MD, and H. G. Adelson. "The Efficacy of Progesterone in Achieving Successful Pregnancy: II. In Women with Pure Luteal Phase Defects." *International Journal of Fertility* 32, no. 2 (1987): 139–41.

Cousens, Gabriel, MD, with Mark Mayell. *Depression-Free for Life*. New York: Harper Collins, 2000.

Curcio, J., D. A. Wollner, J. W. Schmidt, and L. S. Kim. "Is Bio-Identical Hormone Replacement Therapy Safer Than Traditional Hormone Replacement Therapy?: A Critical Appraisal of Cardiovascular Risks in Menopausal Women." *Treatments in Endocrinology* 5, no. 6 (2006): 367–74.

Dach, Jeffrey. *Bioidentical Hormones 101*. Davie, FL: Dach Press, 2012.

Dalton, K., MD. *Depression after Childbirth: How to Recognize, Treat, and Prevent Postnatal Depression*. New York: Oxford University Press, 1989.

Dalton, K., MD, with W. Holton. *Once a Month: Understanding and Treating PMS*. Alameda, CA: Hunter House, Inc., 1999.

Eden J. "Progestins and Breast Cancer." *American Journal of Obstetrics and Gynecology* 188, no. 5 (May 2003): 1123–31.

Edinger, Edward. *Ego and Archetype*. London and Boston: Shambala, 1972.

Evans, Patricia. *Controlling People: How to Recognize, Understand, and Deal with People Who Try to Control You*. Avon, MA: Adams Media, 2002.

Fitzpatrick, L. A., MD, C. Pace, BS, and B. Wiita. "Comparison of Regimens Containing Oral Micronized Progesterone or Medroxyprogesterone Acetate on Quality of Life in Postmenopausal Women: A Cross-Sectional Survey." *Journal of Women's Health and Gender-Based Medicine* 9, no. 6 (2000).

Fournier, A., F. Berrino, E. Riboli, V. Avenel, and F. Clavel-Chapelon. "Breast Cancer Risk in Relation to Different Types of Hormone Replacement Therapy in E3N-EPIC Cohort." *International Journal of Cancer* 114, no. 3 (April 10, 2005): 448–54.

Foy, M. R., J. Xu, X. Xie, R. D. Brinton, R. F. Thompson, and T. W. Berger. "17-Estradiol Enhances NMDA Receptor-Mediated EPSPs and Long-Term Potentiation." *Journal of Neurophysiology* 81 (1999): 925–29.

Gaby, A. R., MD. "Estrogen Replacement Therapy." In *Preventing & Reversing Osteoporosis*. New York: Three Rivers Press, 1994.

Genazzani, J., and B. Nilsen, RD. "Estrogen Regulation of Mitochondrial Function and Impact of the Aging Process. Calcium, Glutamate-Induced Excitotoxicity and Estrogen Induced Neuroprotection." In *Hormone Replacement Therapy and the Brain*, by A. Genazzani. Boca Raton, FL: CRC Press, 2003.

Glenmullen, Joseph. *Prozac Backlash*. New York: Simon and Schuster, 2007.

Graboys, T. B., A. Headley, B. Lown, S. Lampert, and C. M. Blatt. "Results of a Second-Opinion Program for Coronary Artery Bypass Surgery." *Journal of the American Medical Association* 258 (September 1987): 1611–14.

Greenlee, H., Y. Chen, G. C. Kabat, Q. Wang, M. G. Kibriya, I. Gurvich, D. W. Sepkovic, H. L. Bradlow, R. T. Senie, R. M. Santella, and H. Ahsan. "Variants in Estrogen Metabolism and Biosynthesis Genes and Urinary Estrogen Metabolites in Women with a Family History of Breast Cancer." *Breast Cancer Research and Treatment* 102, no. 1 (March 2007): 111–17.

Harding, M. Esther. *Women's Mysteries: Ancient and Modern*. New York: Harper, 1976.

Hargrove, J. T., MD, W. S. Maxson, MD, and A. Colston Wentz, MD. "Absorption of Oral Progesterone Is Influenced by Vehicle and Particle Size." *American Journal of Obstetrics and Gynecology* 161, no. 4 (October 1989): 948–51.

Hargrove, J. T., MD, W. S. Maxson, MD, A. Colston Wentz, MD, and L. S. Burnett, MD. "Menopausal Hormone Replacement Therapy with Continuous Daily Oral Micronized Estradiol and Progesterone." *Obstetrics and Gynecology* 73, no. 4 (April 1989): 606–12.

Head, K. A., ND. "Estriol: Safety and Efficacy." *Alternative Medicine Review* 3, no. 2 (1998): 101–13.

Herzog, Andrew G., M.D. "Progesterone Therapy in Women with Complex Partial and Secondary Generalized Seizures." *Neurology* 45, no. 9 (September 1995).

Hoeller, Stephan. *The Gnostic Jung and the Seven Sermons to the Dead*. Chicago: Theosophical Publishing House, 1982.

Hoffer, Abram. *Adventures in Psychiatry*. Ontario, Canada: KOS Publishing, 2005.

Hotze, Steven. *Hormones, Health, and Happiness*. Houston, TX: Forrest Publishing, 2005.

Hutchinson, Karen. *What Every Woman Needs to Know about Estrogen*. New York: Penguin/Plume, 1997.

Johnson, Robert. *Inner Gold: Understanding Psychological Projection*. Kihei, HI: Koa Books, 2006.

Jung, C. G. *Jung on Active Imagination*. Princeton, NJ: Princeton University Press, 1997.

Klaiber, E. L. *Hormones and the Mind*. New York: Harper Paperbacks, 2002.

Lark, Susan M. *Heavy Menstrual Flow and Anemia*. Berkeley, CA: Third Edition Celestial Arts, 1999.

LeDoux, Joseph. *The Emotional Brain: The Mysterious Underpinnings*. New York: Touchstone, 1996.

———. *Synaptic Self*. New York: Viking, 2004.

Lee, John. *Natural Progesterone: The Multiple Roles of a Remarkable Hormone*. Chicago: Jon Carpenter Publishing, 2001.

Lee, John, and V. Hopkins. *What Your Doctor May Not Tell You about Menopause*. New York: Warner Books, 1996.

Lee, John, D. Zava, and V. Hopkins. *What Your Doctor May Not Tell You about Breast Cancer*. New York: Warner Books, 2002.

Lehninger, Albert L. *Bioenergetics: The Molecular Basis of Biological Energy Transformations*. California: W. A. Benjamin, Inc., 1973.

Levitan, Irwin B., and L. K. Kaczmarek. *The Neuron: Cell and Molecular Biology*. New York: Oxford University Press, 2002.

L'Hermite, M., T. Simoncini, S. Fuller, and A. R. Genazzani. "Could Transdermal Estradiol + Progesterone Be a Safer Postmenopausal HRT? A Review." *Maturitas* 60, no. 3–4 (July–August 2008): 185–201.

Lord, Richard, and J. A. Bralley. *Laboratory Evaluations for Integrative and Functional Medicine*. Duluth, GA: Metametrix Institute, 2008.

Marin, R., B. Guerra, J. G. Hernández-Jiménez, X. L. Kang, J. D. Fraser, F. J. López, and R. Alonso. "Estradiol Prevents Amyloid-Beta Peptide-Induced Cell Death in a Cholinergic Cell Line via Modulation of a Classical Estrogen Receptor." *Neuroscience* 121, no. 4 (2003): 917–26.

McCann, S. E., J. Wactawski-Wende, K. Kufel, J. Olson, B. Ovando, S. N. Kadlubar, W. Davis, L. Carter, P. Muti, P. G. Shields, and J. L. Freudenheim. "Changes in 2-hydroxyestrone and 16{alpha}-hydroxyestrone Metabolism with Flaxseed Consumption: Modification by COMT and CYP1B1 Genotype." *Cancer Epidemiology Biomarkers and Prevention* 16, no. 2 (2007): 256–62.

Meade, Michael. *The Water of Life*. Seattle: Greenfire Press/Mosaic Multicultural Foundation, 2006.

Miller, Karen, and Steven Rogers. *The Estrogen-Depression Connection*. Oakland, CA: New Harbinger, 2007.

Misu, Yoshima, and Yoshio Goshima. *Neurobiology of DOPA as a Neurotransmitter*. Boca Raton, FL: CRC Press, 2006.

Miyagawa, K., J. Rösch, F. Stanczyk, and K. Hermsmeyer. "Medroxyprogesterone Interferes with Ovarian Steroid Protection against Coronary Vasospasm." *Nature Medicine* 3, no. 3 (1997): 324–27.

Mooradian, A. D., J. E. Morley, and S. G. Korenman. "Biological Actions of Androgens." *Endocrine Society* 8, no. 1 (February 1987): 1–28.

Mosby's Drug Consult for Nurses. Waltham, MA: Elsevier, 2006.

Naik, R., S. Nixon, A. Lopes, K. Godfrey, M. H. Hatem, and J. M. Monaghan. "A Randomized Phase II Trial of Indole-3-Carbinol in the Treatment of Vulvar Intraepithelial Neoplasia." *International Journal of Gynecological Cancer* 16, no. 2 (2006): 786–90.

Nelson, David, and M. M. Cox. *Lehninger: Principles of Biochemistry*. New York: Worth, 2000.

Newbold, H. L. *Mega-Nutrients for Your Nerves*. New York: Wyden, 1975.
Northrup, Christiane. *Women's Bodies, Women's Wisdom*. New York: Bantam, 1995.
Perlmutter, David. BrainRecovery.com. Naples, FL: Perlmutter Health Center, 2000.
Pert, Candace. *Molecules of Emotion: The Science behind Mind-Body Medicine*. New York: Scribner, 2007.
Pfaff, Donald. *Drive: Neurobiological and Molecular Mechanisms of Sexual Motivation*. Cambridge, MA: MIT Press, 1999.
Pfaff, Donald, M. I. Phillips, and R. T. Rubin. *Principles of Hormone/Behavior Relations*. Waltham, MA: Elsevier Press, 2004.
Raff, Jeffrey. *Jung and the Alchemical Imagination*. York Beach, ME: Nicolas-Hays, 2000.
Rasgon, N. L. *The Effects of Estrogen on Brain Function*. Baltimore: Johns Hopkins University Press, 2006.
Raz, R., MD, and W. E. Stamm, MD. "A Controlled Trial of Intravaginal Estriol in Postmenopausal Women with Recurrent Urinary Tract Infections." *New England Journal of Medicine* 329, no. 11 (September 1993): 753–56.
Rinzler, Carol Ann. *Estrogen and Breast Cancer: A Warning to Women*. Alameda, CA: Hunter House Books, 1996.
Rogers, Sherry. *Depression: Cured at Last!* New York: Prestige Publishing, 1996.
Sapolsky, Robert. *Why Zebras Don 't Get Ulcers*. New York: Freeman, 2000.
Schachter, Michael. *What Your Doctor May Not Tell You about Depression*. New York: Warner Books, 2006.
Shepherd, Gordon. *Synaptic Organization of the Brain*. New York: Oxford University Press, 1998.
Sismondo, Sergio, and Mathieu Doucet. "Publication Ethics and the Ghost Management of Medical Publication." *Bioethics* 24, no. 6 (July 2010): 273–83.
Skoog, Douglas A. *Principles of Instrumental Analysis*. New York: Saunders College Publishing, 1992.
Smith, S. S. *Neurosteroid Effects in the Central Nervous System: The Role of the GABA-A Receptor*. Boca Raton, FL: CRC Press, 2003.
Sowers, M. R., S. Crawford, D. McConnell, J. R. Randolph Jr., E. B. Gold, M. K. Wilkin, and B. Lasley. "Selected Diet and Lifestyle Factors Are Associated with Estrogen Metabolites in Multiracial/Ethnic Population of Women." *Journal of Nutrition* 136, no. 6 (2006): 1588–95.
Sowers, M. R., D. McConnell, M. Jannausch, A. G. Buyuktur, M. Hochberg, and D. A. Jamadar. "Estradiol and Its Metabolites and Their Association with Knee Arthritis." *Arthritis Rheum* 54, no. 8 (2006): 2481–87.
Sowers, M. R., A. L. Wilson, S. R. Kardia, J. Chu, and D. S. McConnell. "CYP1A1 and CYP1B1 Polymorphisms and Their Association with Estradiol and Estrogen Metabolites in Women Who Are Premenopausal and Perimenopausal." *American Journal of Medicine* 119, 9, Supplement 1 (2006): S44–51.
Swaneck, G. E., and J. Fishman. "Covalent Binding of the Endogenous Estrogen 16 Alpha-Hydroxyestrone to Estradiol Receptor in Human Breast Cancer Cells." *Proceedings of the National Academy of Science USA* 85, no. 21 (1988): 7831–35.
Taylor, Maida, MD. "'Bioidentical' Estrogens: Hope or Hype?" *Sexuality, Reproduction, and Menopause* 3, no. 2 (October 2005): 68–71.
Vliet, Elizabeth Lee. *It's My Ovaries, Stupid!* New York: Scribner, 2003.
———. *The Savvy Woman's Guide to Testosterone*. Arizona: Her Place Press, 2005.
von Bohlen und Halbach, O., and R. Dermietzel. *Neurotransmitters and Neuromodulators*. Weinheim, Germany: Wiley-VCH, 2001.
von Franz, Marie L. *The Psychological Meaning of Redemption Motifs in Fairy Tales*. Toronto, Canada: Inner City Books, 1980.
Warga, Claire. *Menopause and the Mind*. New York: Free Press, 1999.
Watson, James. *DNA: The Secret of Life*. New York: Knopf, 2003.
Werbach, Melvyn. *Healing through Nutrition*. New York: HarperCollins, 1993.
———. *Nutritional Influences on Mental Illness*. Tarzana, CA: Third Line Press, 1991.
Woodman, Marion. *The Pregnant Virgin*. Toronto, Canada: Inner City Books, 1985.

Woolley, C. S., and B. S. McEwen. "Roles of Estradiol and Progesterone in Regulation Hippocampal Dendritic Spine Density during Estrous Cycle in the Rat." *Journal of Comparative Neurology* 336, no. 2 (1993): 293–306.

Wright, J. V., MD, B. Schliesman, MCT, and L. Robinson, MCT. "Comparative Measurements of Serum Estriol, Estradiol, and Estrone in Non-Pregnant, Premenopausal Women: A Preliminary Investigation." *Alternative Medicine Review* 4, no. 4 (1999): 266–70.

Wu, W. H., Y. P. Kang, N. H. Wang, H. J. Jou, and T. A. Wang. "Sesame Ingestion Affects Sex Hormones, Antioxidant Status, and Blood Lipids in Postmenopausal Women." *Journal of Nutrition* 136, no. 5 (2006): 1270–75.

ONLINE LINKS

Barbour, Ginny. "Ghostauthors, Ghost Management and the Manipulation of Medical Research." CommitteeonPublicationEthics.com, http://publicationethics.org/blogs/ghostauthors-ghost-management-and-manipulation-medical-research.

Cirigliano, M., MD, FACP. "Bioidentical Hormone Therapy: A Review of the Evidence." *Journal of Women's Health* 16, no. 5 (2007): 600–31. University of Pennsylvania School of Medicine, Philadelphia, Pennsylvania, http://www.solaltech.com/doctors/3/Bioidentical%20Hormone%20Therapy--%20Cirigliano.pdf.

Collier, Roger. "Prevalence of Ghostwriting Spurs Calls for Transparency." *Canadian Medical Association Journal* 181, no. 8 (2009), http://www.cmaj.ca/earlyreleases/9sept09_ghostwriting.dtl.

Drug Industry Document Archive (DIDA), http://dida.library.ucsf.edu/documents.jsp. The Drug Industry Document Archive (DIDA) contains drug company documents and external resources about drug industry clinical trials, publication of results, pricing, marketing, relations with physicians, and involvement in continuing medical education.

Flanagin, Annette, Lisa A. Carey, Phil B. Fontanarosa, Stephanie G. Phillips, Brian P. Pace, George L. Lundberg, and Drummond Rennie. "Prevalence of Articles with Honorary Authors and Ghost Authors in Peer-Reviewed Medical Journals." *Journal of the American Medical Association* 280, no. 3 (1998): 222–24, http://jama.jamanetwork.com/article.aspx?articleid=187772.

Fournier, Agnès, F. Berrino, and F. Clavel-Chapelon. "Unequal Risks for Breast Cancer Associated with Different Hormone Replacement Therapies: Results from the E3N Cohort Study." *Breast Cancer Research and Treatment* 107, no. 1 (January 2008), http://www.ncbi.nlm.nih.gov/pmc/articles/PMC2211383/.

Fugh-Berman, Adriane, and Jenna Bythrow. "Bioidentical Hormones for Menopausal Hormone Therapy: Variation on a Theme." *Journal of General Intern Medicine* 22, no. 7 (July 2007): 1030–34, http://www.ncbi.nlm.nih.gov/pmc/articles/PMC2219716/.

Grassley, Charles E. "Ghostwriting in Medical Literature." Minority Staff Report, 111th Congress, U.S. Senate Committee on Finance, June 24, 2010, http://grassley.senate.gov/about/upload/Senator-Grassley-Report.pdf.

Holtorf, Kent, MD. "The Bioidentical Hormone Debate: Are Bioidentical Hormones (Estradiol, Estriol, and Progesterone) Safer or More Efficacious Than Commonly Used Synthetic Versions in Hormone Replacement Therapy?" PostgraduateMedicine.com, http://www.postgradmed.com/index.php?article=1949.

Hotze, Steven F., MD, and Donald P. Ellsworth, MD. "Point/Counterpoint: The Case for Bioidentical Hormones." *Journal of American Physicians and Surgeons* 13, no. 2 (Summer 2008), 43, http://www.jpands.org/vol13no2/hotze.pdf.

Jirik, Kate. "How Great Researchers Get By-lines, Get Paid, and Get Medicine in Trouble." Medicine and Business, BioethicsForum.com, December 28, 2006, http://www.thehastingscenter.org/Bioethicsforum/Post.aspx?id=326.

Kotur, P. F. "Transgression in Scientific Communication." *Indian Journal of Anaesthetics* 54, no. 1 (January–February 2010), 2–4, http://www.ncbi.nlm.nih.gov/pmc/articles/ PMC2876906/.

Lacasse, Jeffrey R., and Jonathan Leo. "Ghostwriting at Elite Academic Medical Centers in the United States," *PLoS Medicine* 7, no. 2 (2010): 1–4, http://www.plosmedicine.org/ article/info:doi%2F10.1371%2Fjournal.pmed.1000230.

Moisse, Katie. "Ghostbusters: Authors of a New Study Propose a Strict Ban on Medical Ghostwriting." ScientificAmerican.com, February 4, 2010, http://www.scientificamerican. com/article.cfm?id=ghostwriter-science-industry. A scientist who takes credit as an author for an article secretly written by a pharmaceutical company should face punishment like any other plagiarist. Lacasse and Leo even recommend that scientists who have participated in ghostwriting in the past should confess and that their ghostwritten papers be reevaluated and even retracted if appropriate.

Moskowitz, Deborah, ND. "A Comprehensive Review of the Safety and Efficacy of Bioidentical Hormones for the Management of Menopause and Related Health Risks." *Alternative Medicine Review* 11, no. 3 (2006): 208–23, http://www.thorne.com/altmedrev/.fulltext/11/3/208.pdf.

"Public Disclosure and Authorship." Pfizer.com, http://www.pfizer.com/research/research_ clinical_trials/registration_disclosure_authorship.jsp. Authors must also acknowledge individuals who provide editorial support and disclose the funding source. For Pfizer-sponsored studies, the fact that the study was funded by Pfizer must be disclosed.

Rosenberg, Martha. "Pfizer's Ghostwritten Journal Articles Are Still Standing, Still Bogus." AltheoNews.com, February 23, 2010, http://alethonews.wordpress.com/2010/02/23/pfizers-ghostwritten-journal-articles-are-still-standing-still-bogus/.

Schwartz, Erika, and Kent Holtorf. "Hormones in Wellness and Disease Prevention: Common Practices, Current State of the Evidence, and Questions for the Future." *Primary Care: Clinics in Office Practice* 35 (2008), http://www.carrollwoodpharmacy.com/ carrollwoodpharmacy/Bio/Bio.pdf.

Schwartz, Erika, Kent Holtorf, and David Brownstein. "The Truth about Hormone Therapy." WallStreetJournal.com, March 16, 2009, http://online.wsj.com/article/ SB123717056802137143.html.

She, Jin-Xiong, T. M. Ellis, S. B. Brian et al. "Heterophile Antibodies Segregate in Families and Are Associated with Protection from Type 1 Diabetes." *Proceedings of the National Academy of Science* 96, no. 14 (July 1999), http://www.ncbi.nlm.nih.gov/pmc/articles/ PMC22197?tool=pmcentrez.

Singer, Natasha. "Medical Papers by Ghostwriters Pushed Therapy." NewYorkTimes.com, August 4, 2009, http://www.nytimes.com/2009/08/05/health/research/05ghost.html?_r=1& ref=health.

———. "Senator Moves to Block Medical Ghostwriting." NewYorkTimes.com, August 18, 2009, http://www.nytimes.com/2009/08/19/health/research/19ethics.html?pagewanted=2. One of the authors discussed in DesignWrite documents is Dr. Michelle P. Warren, a professor of obstetrics and gynecology at Columbia. Her article was published in *American Journal of Obstetrics and Gynecology* in 2004, when women feared that Wyeth's brand of hormone drugs could be causing particular problems.

Walker-Journey, Jennifer. "Ghostwritten Medical Journal Articles about HRT Should Be Retracted." RightingJustice.com, February 9, 2010, http://www.hrt-legal.com/news/2010/ 02/09/ghostwritten-medical-journal-articles-about-hrt-should-be-retracted/.

Wilson, Duff. "Drug Maker Said to Pay Ghostwriters for Journal Articles." NewYorkTimes.com, December 12, 2008, http://www.nytimes.com/2008/12/12/business/13wyeth. html?_r=1&scp=2&sq=wyeth&st=cse.

Wilson, Duff, and Natasha Singer. "Ghostwriting Is Called Rife in Medical Journals." NewYorkTimes.com, September 10, 2009, http://www.nytimes.com/2009/09/11/business/ 11ghost.html.

INDEX

ABOUT THE AUTHORS

Phyllis J. Bronson, PhD, is a research scientist, biochemist, and clinician who has studied the biological impact of molecules on mood and emotion. Bronson has taught neuroscience and conducted hormonal research at the University of Denver and has been a faculty member of the American Academy of Environmental Medicine and the International Society for Orthomolecular Medicine. She was a consultant at the Salpêtrière Hospital in Paris, and was on a task force studying women's mood issues in the military. Bronson lectures frequently throughout the country, and her work has appeared in leading professional journals. She is now president of Biochemical Consulting Company and The Biochemical Research Foundation.

Rebecca Bronson earned a PhD in biochemistry from Boston University and worked for several years at the Shriners Burn Institute in Boston before moving into Research and Development at several different biotechnology companies. After a number of years in industry, she left the field of research science to pursue her two passions—writing and teaching Yoga. She has written several science articles for teens published in *Odyssey* Magazine and is currently managing a Yoga studio and teaching Yoga.